Strictly Curls

A Step-by-Step Guide to Styling Curly Hair

by
Nicole Siri

www.strictlycurls.com

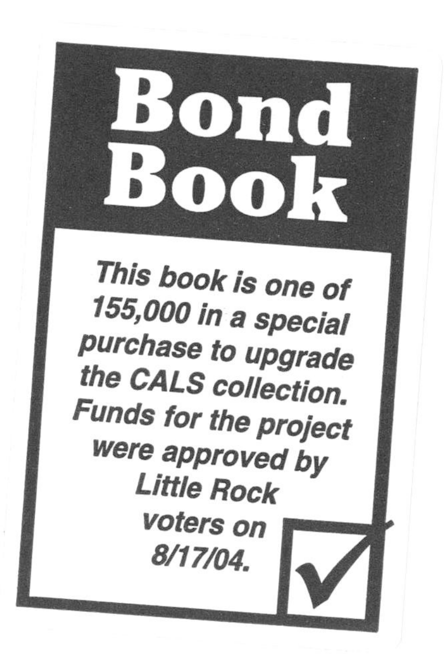

Strictly Curls: A Step-by-Step Guide to Styling Curly Hair
by Nicole Siri

www.strictlycurls.com

Editor: Saranne Fosseman Miller
Cover photograph and all interior photographs are by Jenny Schomaker.

Design: Janet Dell Russell Johnson

ISBN 0-9763506-4-5

Printed and bound in the United States of America.

Acknowledgements

I would like to take this opportunity to show my appreciation to all those who have made this book a reality. I am forever grateful to my loving Heavenly Father for the talents He has blessed me with and the ability to create this book.

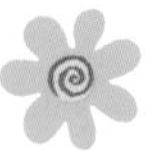

I thank my family, especially my husband, Garrett, for all his support, advice and love.

Many thanks to Jenny Schomaker for her "Eye" in creating the kind of pictures I was looking for, for the many hours she spent in helping me decide the perfect picture for each look, and for being such an insightful and talented photographer and the best sister ever.

Special thanks go to Janet Dell Russell Johnson, responsible for the creative layout of this book. Her artistic flair and professionalism made my visions come to life.

Saranne Fosseman Miller provided valued assistance in preparing this text for print. Without her, I'm afraid only a small percentage of people could have followed my writing. Thanks go as well to China Enright for looking over this text and giving her valued input.

Many thanks to all my family, friends and clients for their thoughts and encouragement.

Finally, I'm grateful to all the curly-haired models who took time out of their busy lives and patiently posed for step-by-step pictures without complaining.
Models printed: Alex, Alina, Ashley, Inna, Jemma, Jessica, Jill, Martha, Saranne, Sue, Quinn.
Make-up for Jemma, Quinn, Inna and Saranne: Nicole Lunetta.

Embrace your curls!

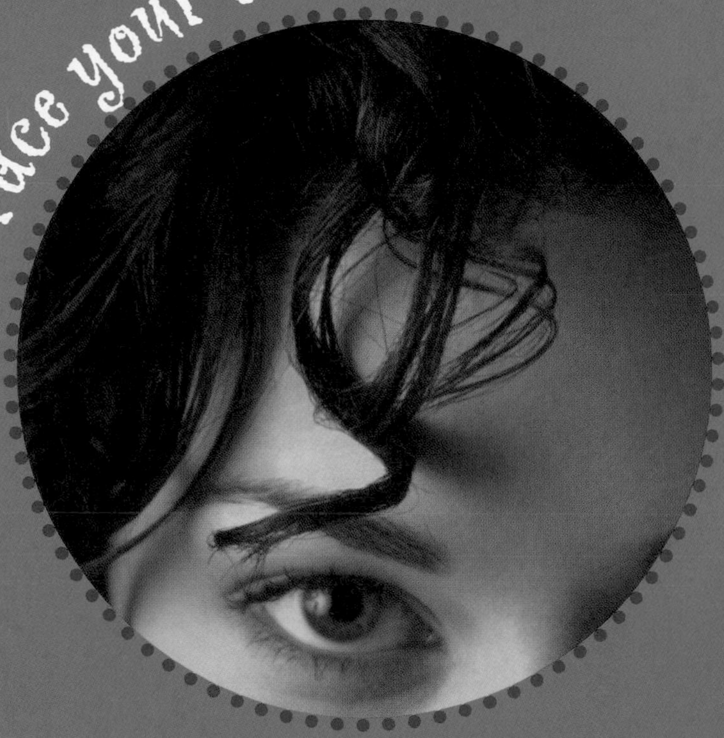

Contents

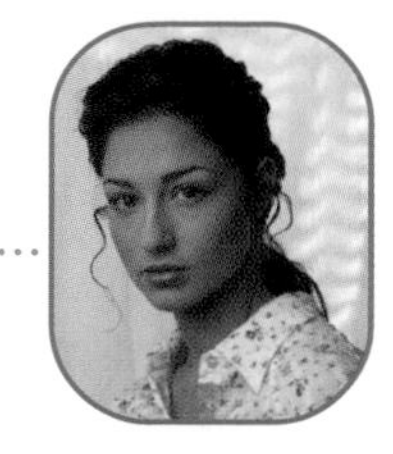

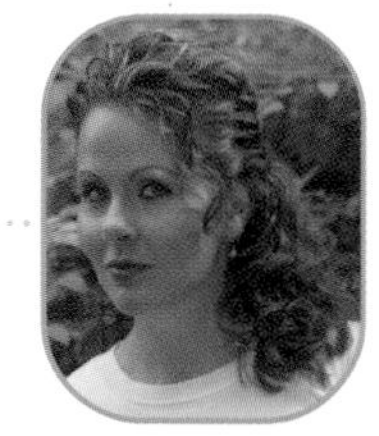

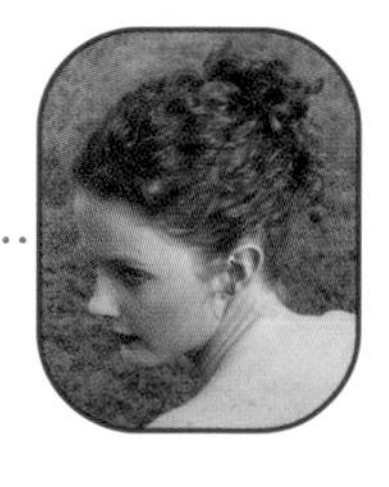

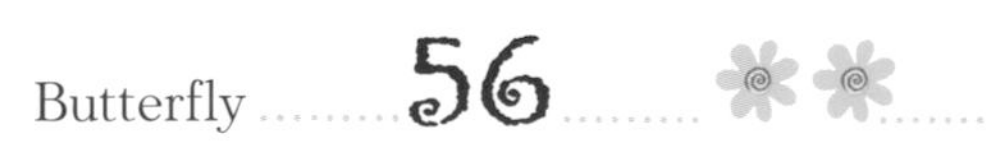

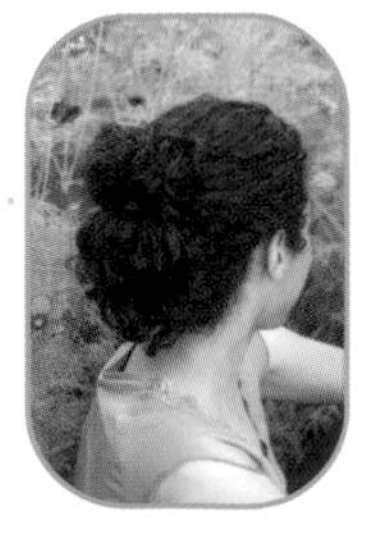

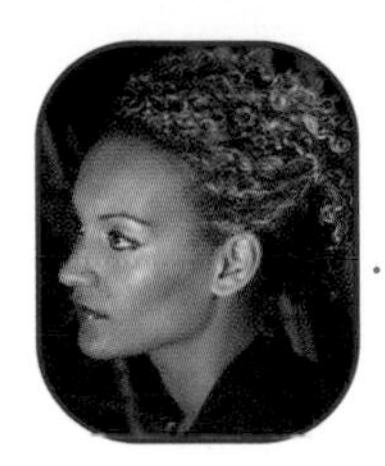

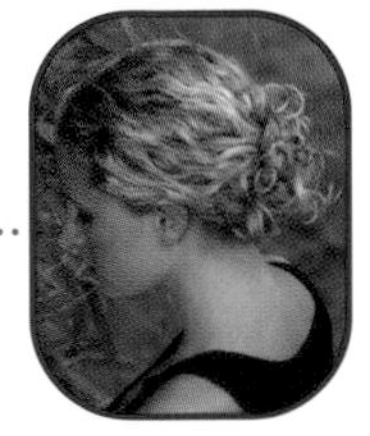

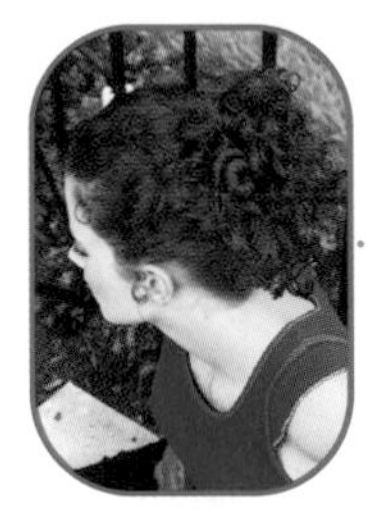

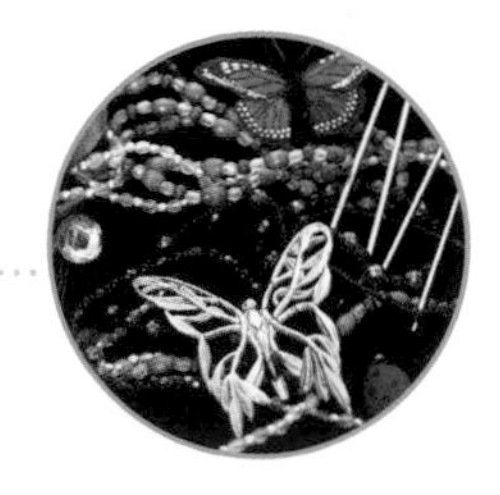

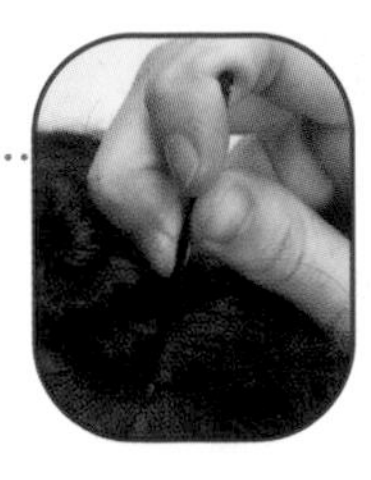

Introduction

Greetings!

I have been a part of the hair industry as a stylist for about a decade. I love meeting new people and helping them enjoy their hair. A few years ago I had the honor of meeting a wonderful lady who introduced me to her philosophy of curly hair. With this new-found enthusiasm for curls, my passion for curly hair grew. While cutting my clients' hair, they would express to me their frustrations and concerns with their curly hair. I heard time and again "I have long, pretty hair but I don't know what to do with it." From my short-haired clients I heard, "I would grow my hair out if I knew what to do with it." So, here it is; everyone who has found themselves saying statements like these, here is a remedy for your worries.

"Strictly Curls" is the solution for all curly-haired women who don't know what to do with their hair. This book is intended to give step-by-step instruction on styling curly hair up. Each style has easy to follow instructions with detailed pictures for each step. There are tips and notes throughout the book, as well as a series of specialty sections in the back. Each look comes with an ability scale. This scale is noted at the top of each different look by showing flowers in the light colored oval. One flower indicates easy—easy in terms of few steps and minimal bobby pinning. Two flowers indicates moderate level of ability; you may need a little hair know-how for these looks. These styles use more bobby pins. I strongly encourage taking a look at the bobby-pinning section of this book (p.86) and practicing the securing techniques before attempting some of these styles. Once you have bobby pinning down, any look is possible. For those of you who can style your hair with ease, you will breeze through the easy and moderate styles. I believe you will enjoy the challenge that comes with the styles indicated by three flowers. These styles require understanding of your hair and the art of placing and securing your hair.

I hope you will find this book informative and useful as a source to draw upon day after day. The way I look at it, you have been blessed with beautiful hair for a lifetime; you might as well learn how to style it. Be patient and remember practice makes perfect!

Nicole Siri

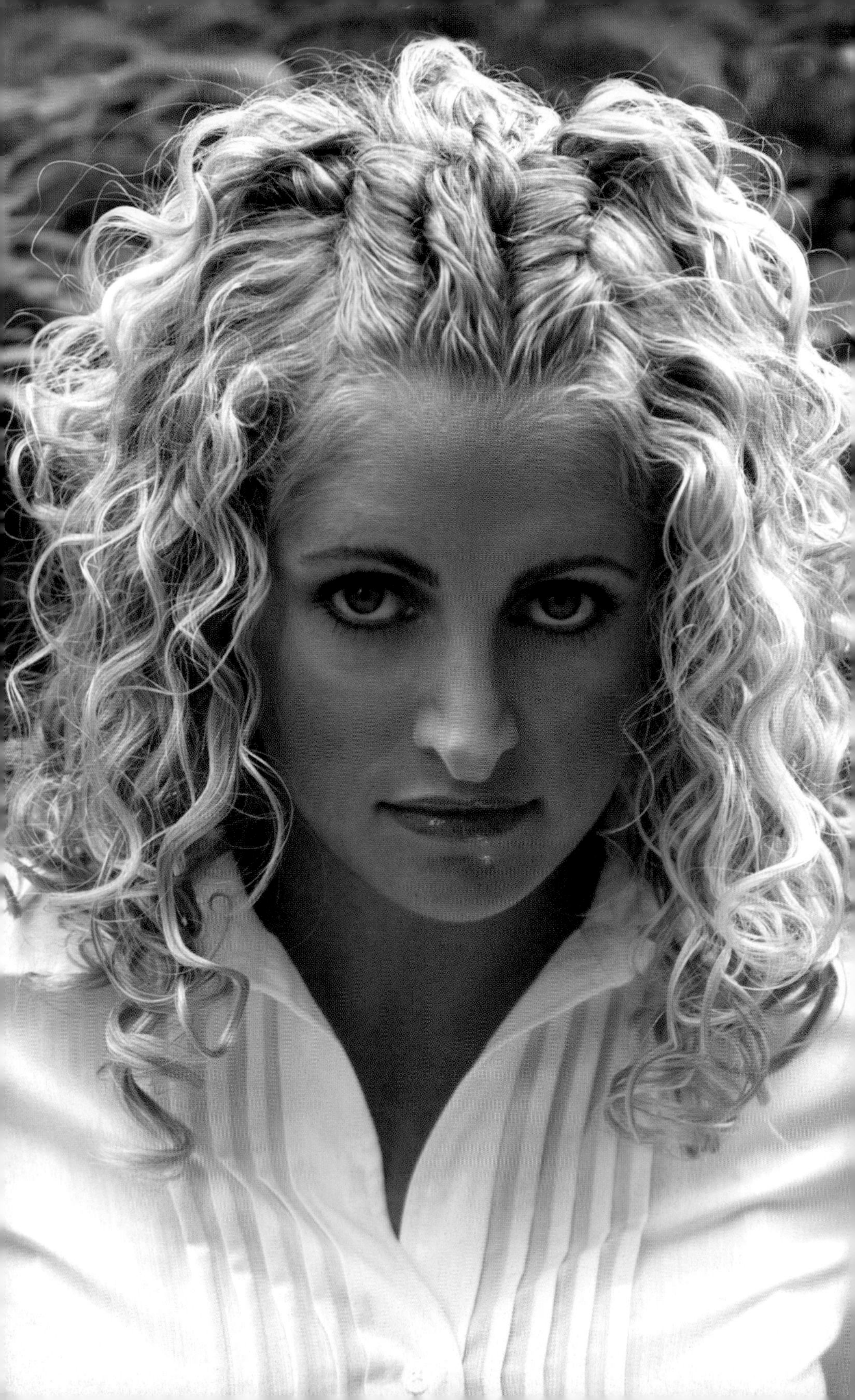

Twist Back

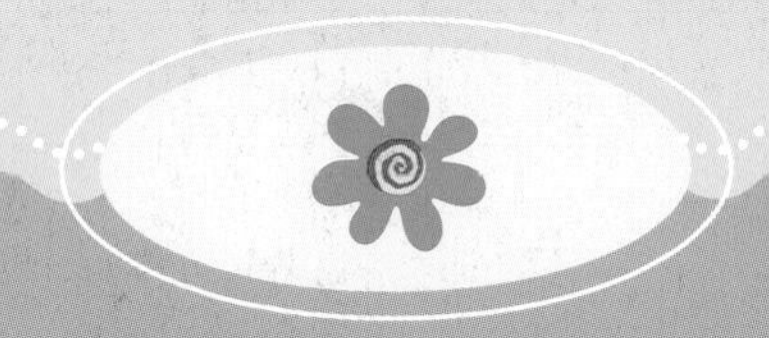

For hair three inches in length or longer.

For some of you, second-day hair is your best hair day. This look is great because you can get the fringe out of the way and still show off your beautiful curls.

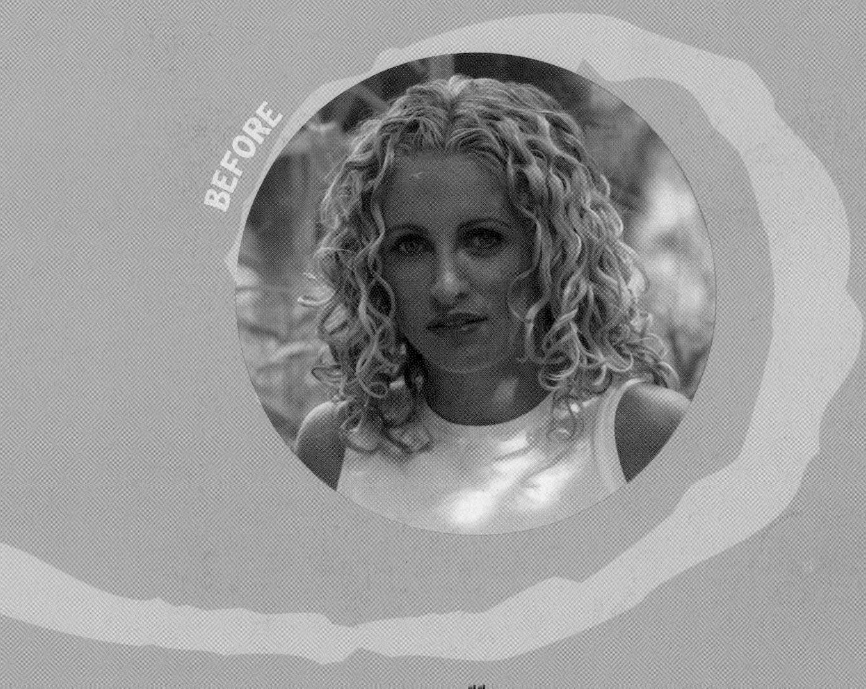

1

Step 1: Gather a one-inch by two-inch section of hair at the brow of your hair line in the center of your head just above your forehead. Twist hair toward the crown of your head.

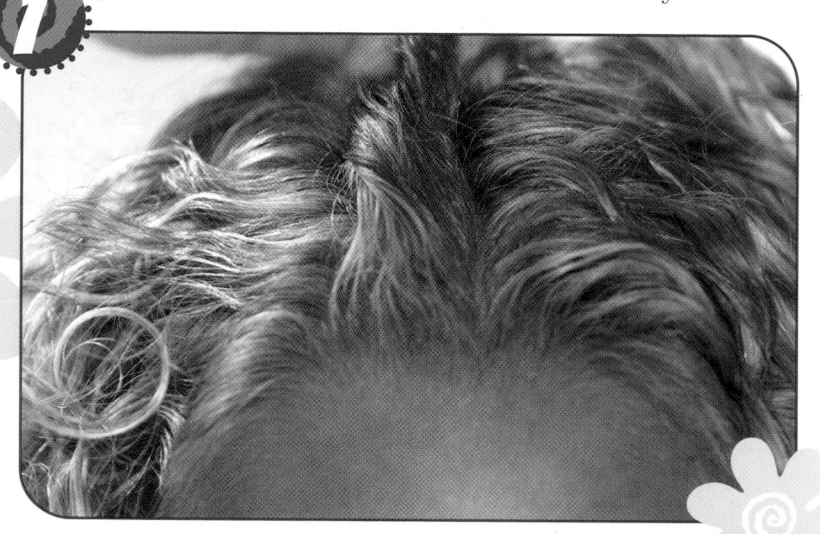

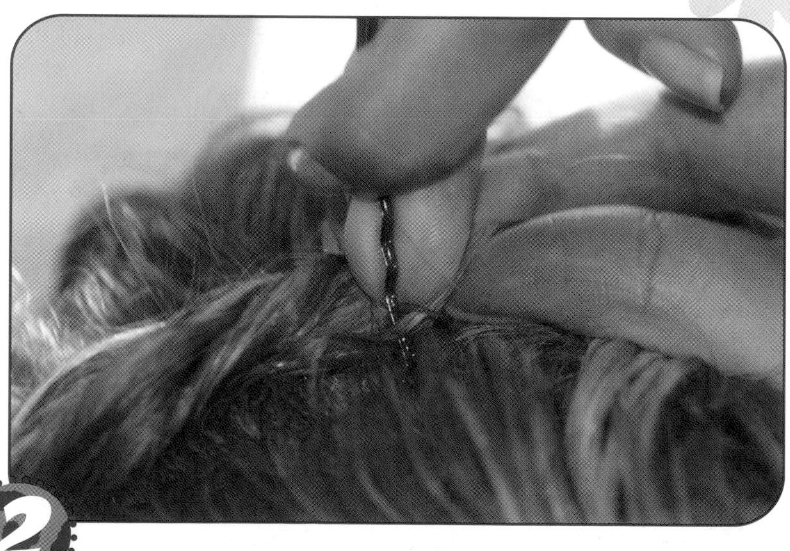

2

Step 2: Secure the twist with a bobby pin. When pinning, straddle your twist with the bobby pin positioning one leg of the pin on either side of the twist. Gently press the bobby pin straight down to the scalp and then push the pin forward and in through the twist, hiding the bobby pin within the hair of the twist.

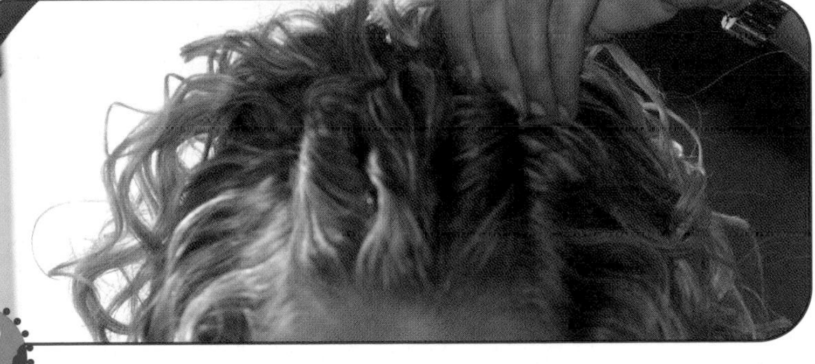

Step 3: Follow Steps 1 and 2, gathering portions of equal sized hair on either side of the existing center twist. Complete one twist to the left of the center and a third twist to the right. Secure the twists as described in Step 2.

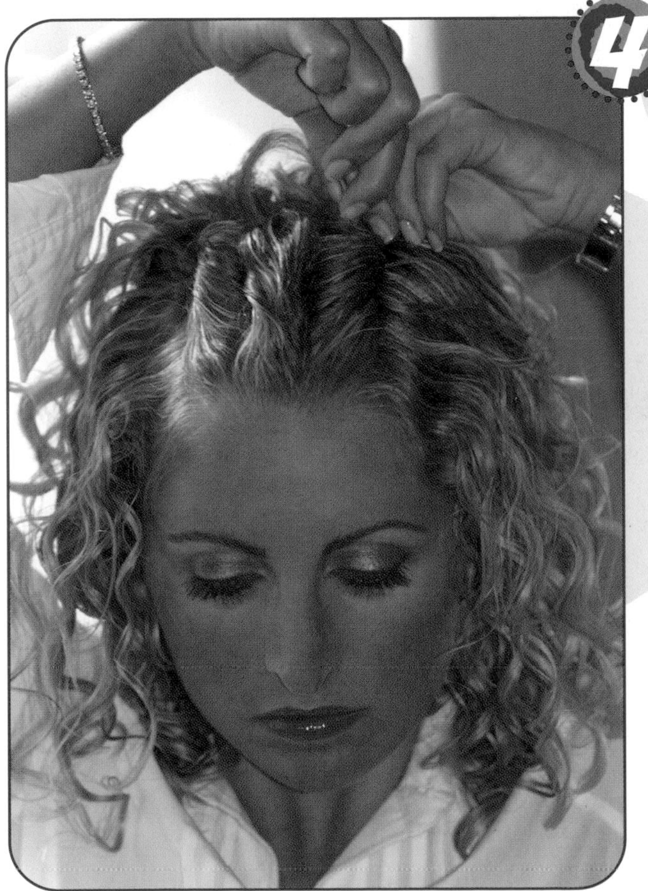

Step 4: Your twist back is complete. Fluff your curls and you are ready for anything that may come your way!

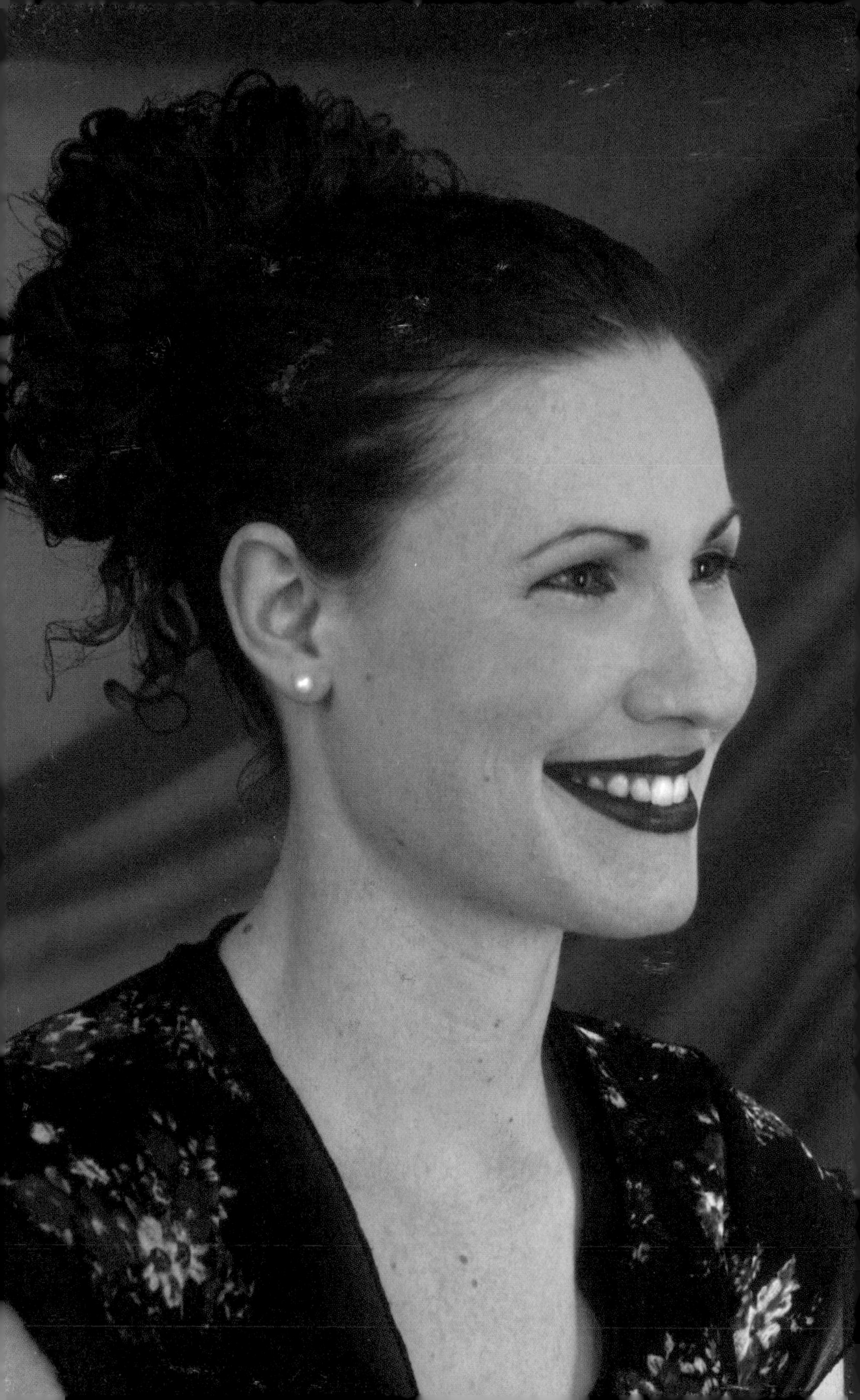

Aphrodite

For shoulder length hair or longer. Can be performed on layered hair as well

With roses to accentuate it, this Goddess of Love style is easy to dress up for a romantic evening. Unadorned, it can be worn around the office or home with equal grace and ease.

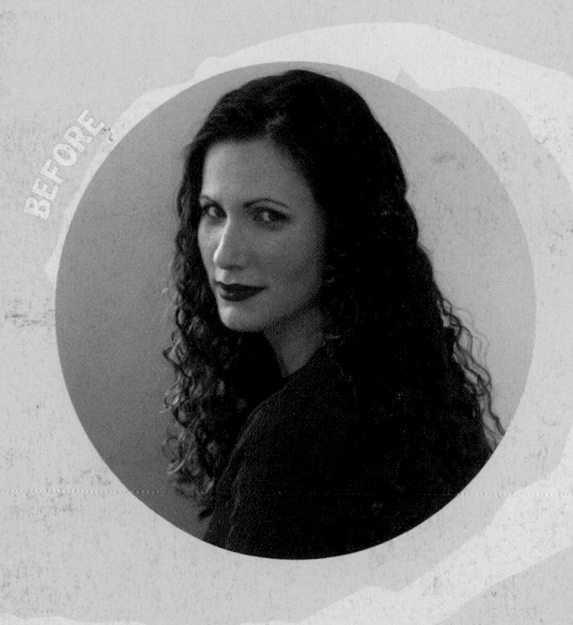

Step 1: Pull hair into a ponytail at the crown of your head and secure with a scrunchy (cloth covered elastic). Wrap the scrunchy several times around the ponytail.

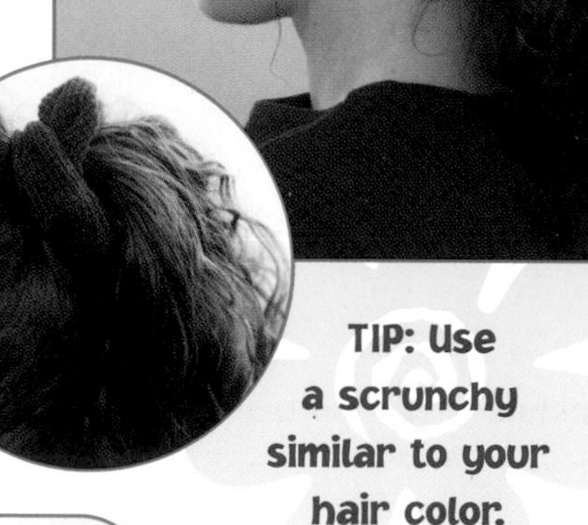

TIP: Use a scrunchy similar to your hair color.

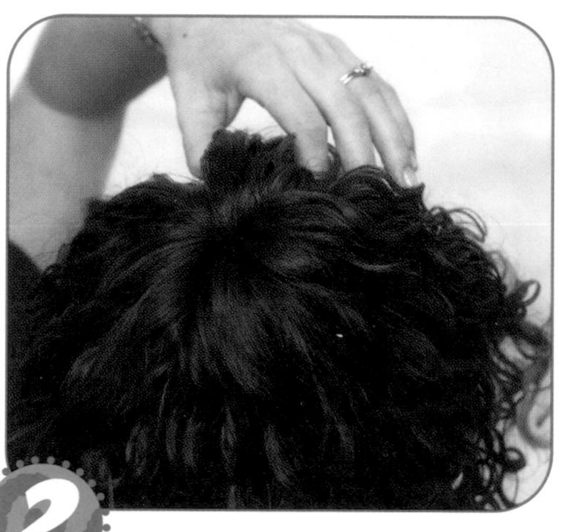

Step 2: Holding head upright, evenly disperse hair over the scrunchy so that the scrunchy is completely covered and hidden by hair.

Step 3: Lift a two-inch section of the dispersed hair from the front of the ponytail and hold in one hand.

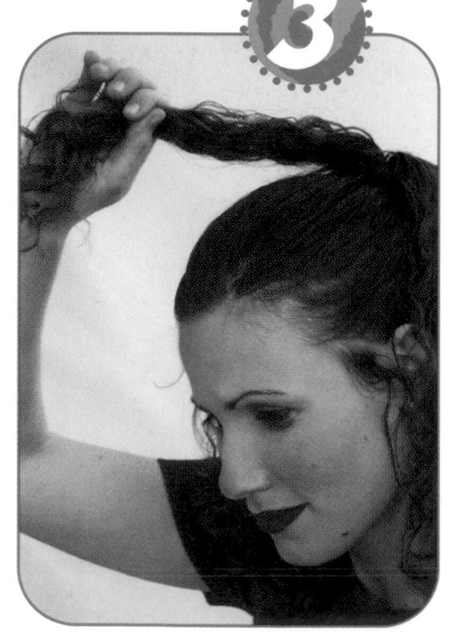

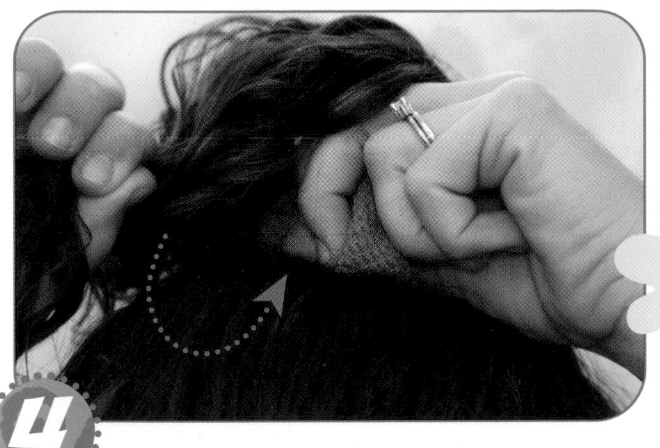

Step 4: Using your free hand, separate a single band from the scrunchy and pull it away from the base of the ponytail. Tuck the two-inch section of hair under the scrunchy from the bottom so that the middle section of hair is held in the scrunchy with the ends of the section of hair sticking out from the bottom.

Step 5: The first tuck is complete. Work around your head in the same manner dividing hair into equal sections and tucking each section of hair into the band of the scrunchy.

Note: The thickness of your hair will determine the number of sections you use for this style. For thicker hair, additional sections of hair may be tucked into the scrunchy.

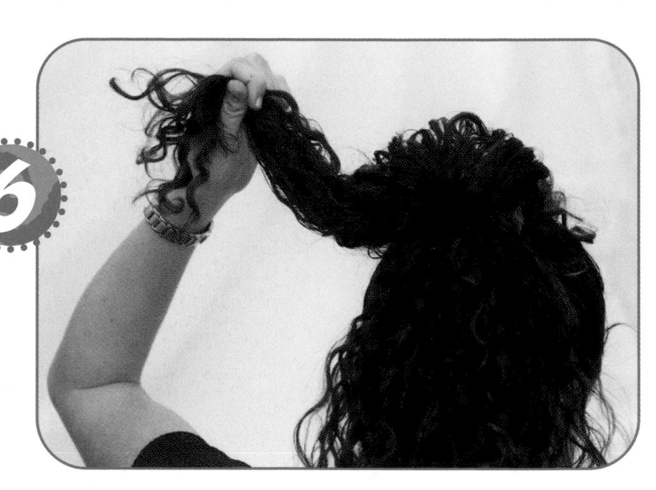

Step 6:
Second tuck position.

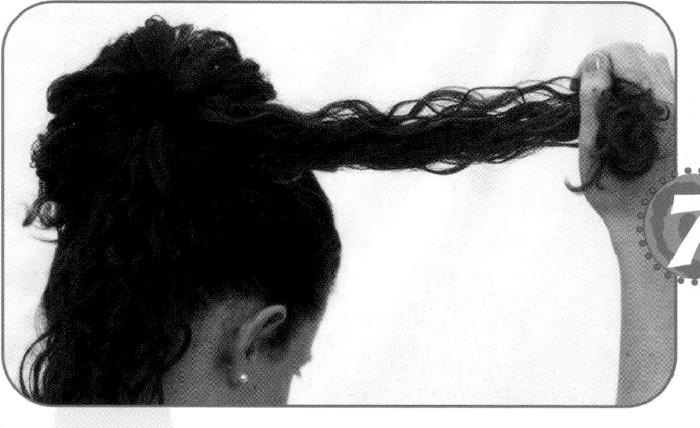

Step 7:
Third tuck is completed.

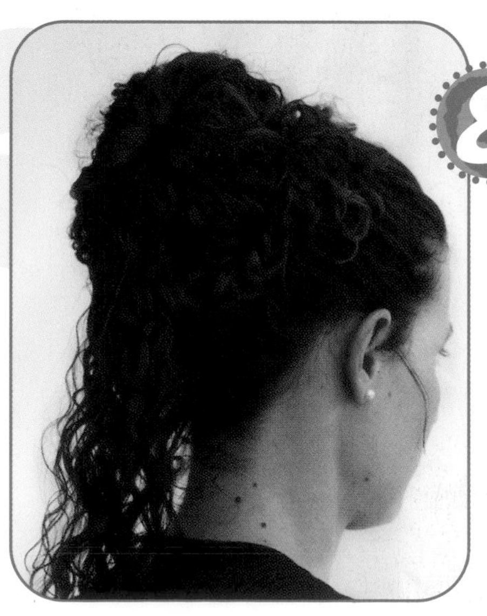

Step 8:
The final section of hair is ready to be tucked into the scrunchy.

Step 9: The style is complete with the final tuck in place.

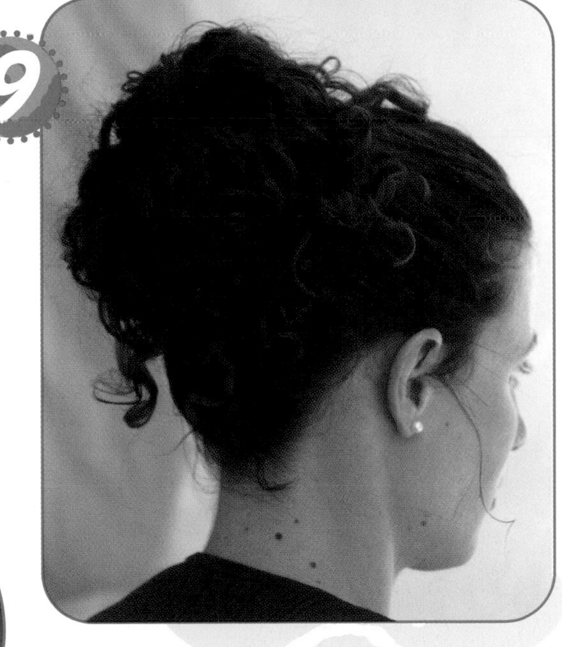

TIP: Enhance the style with flowers or accessories of your choice for a night out.

Worn with everyday fashion, Aphrodite is a versatile style.

TIP: Loosely braiding the sections of hair prior to the tucking process creates another unique look.

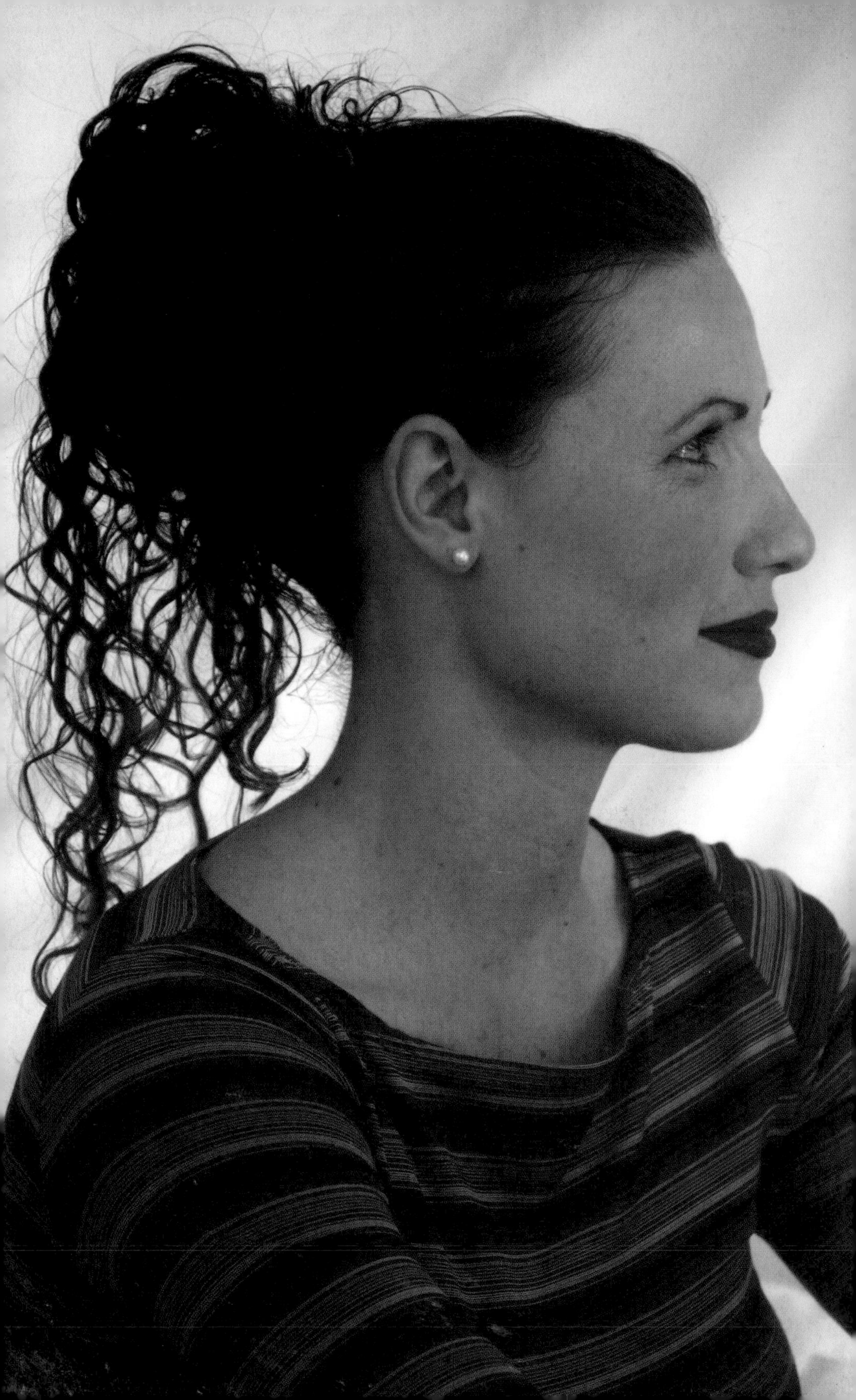

Hestia

For shoulder length hair or longer. Can be performed on layered hair as well

Inspired by the Goddess of Hearth and Home. This style is great for a day of errands and prancing around town. While getting the shopping done you'll look fun and energized.

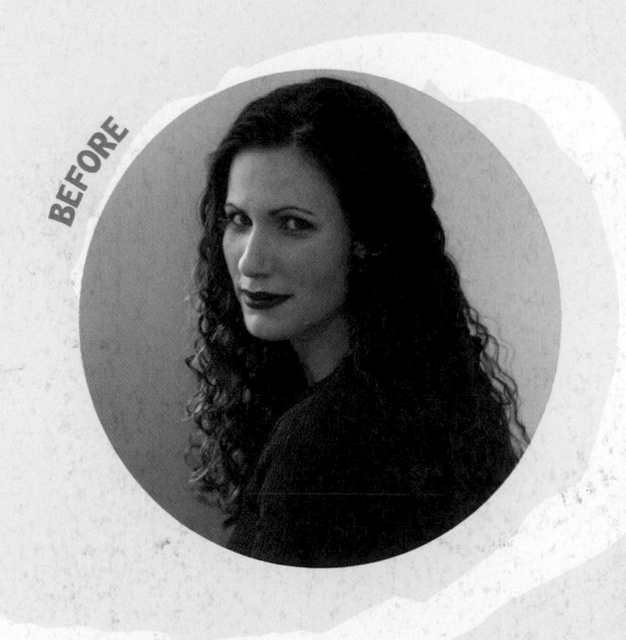

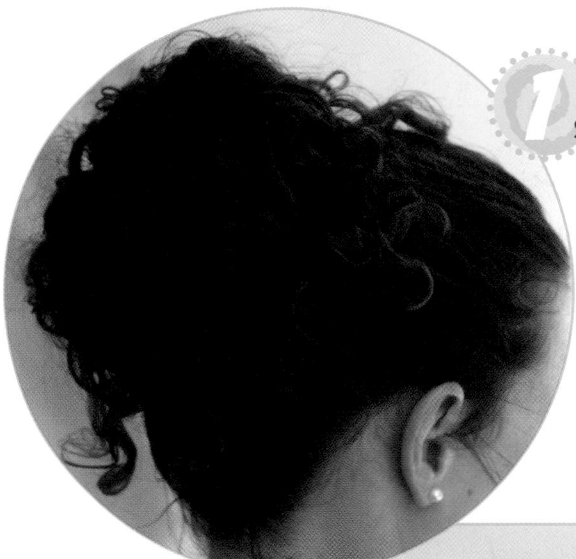

Step 1: You will first need to create the Aphrodite base, by following steps 1 through 9 on pages 16-19.

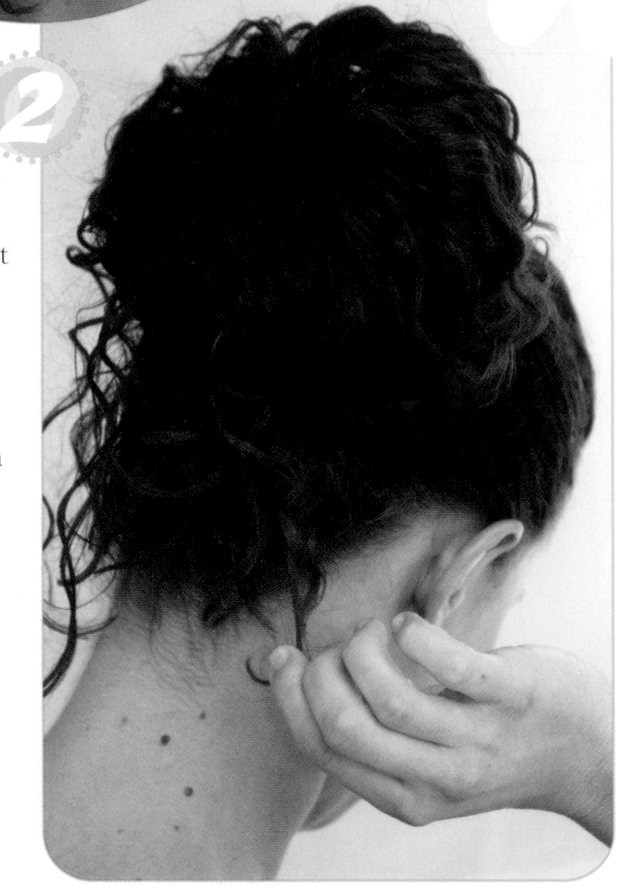

Step 2: Carefully pull on a curl from the perimeter of the style to make it longer. Complete this task on all sections of hair, gently pulling on the loose hair from the center of the style. The length of hair is based on your preference. Balancing the lengths of curls establishes the final look.

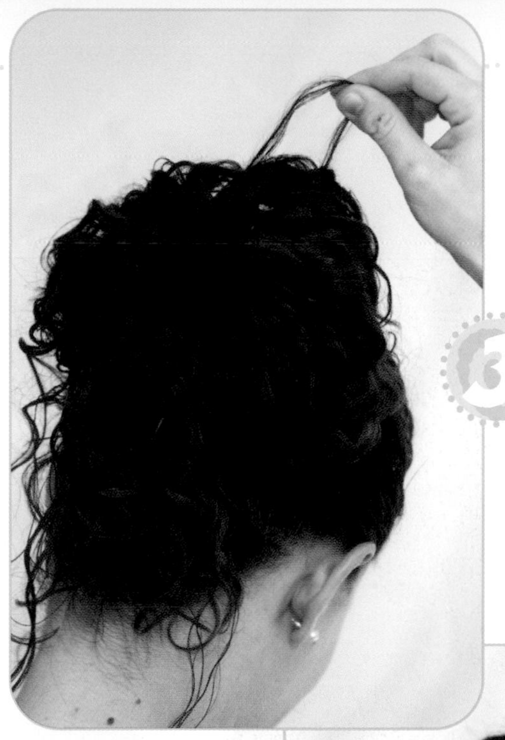

Step 3: Gently cascade small amounts of the sectioned hair over the style.

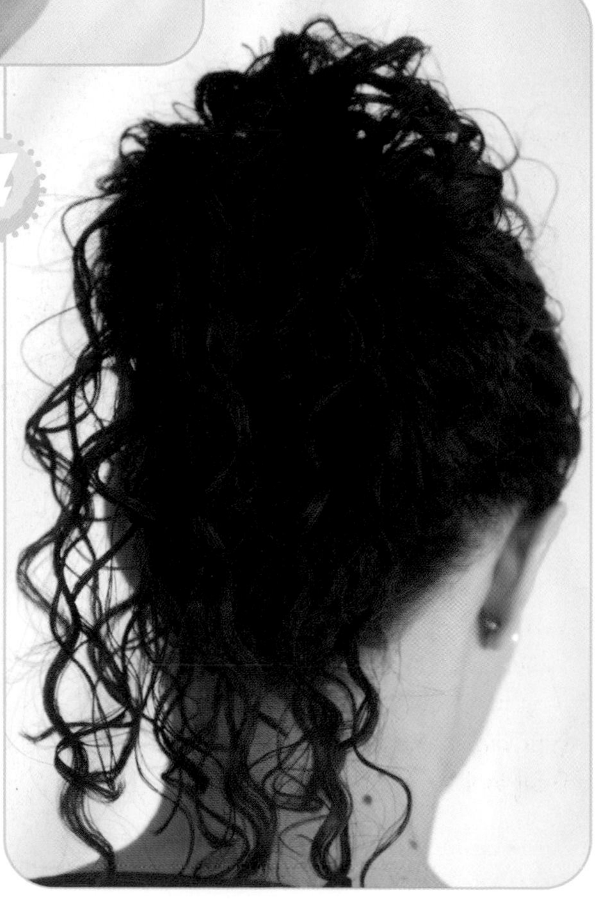

Step 4: Your look is complete. This style can be finished using a curling iron on the sectioned pieces of hair if needed.

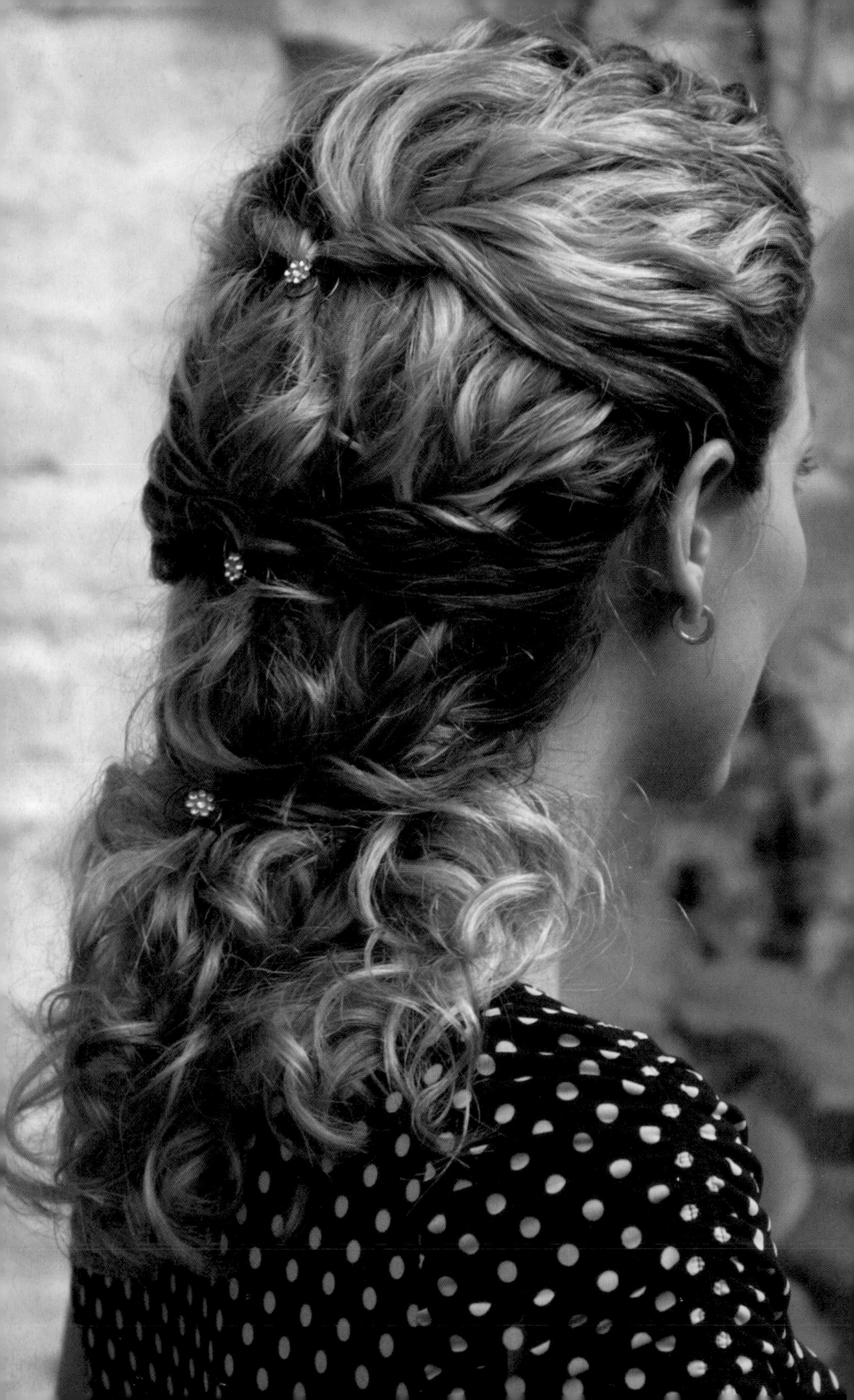

Victorian

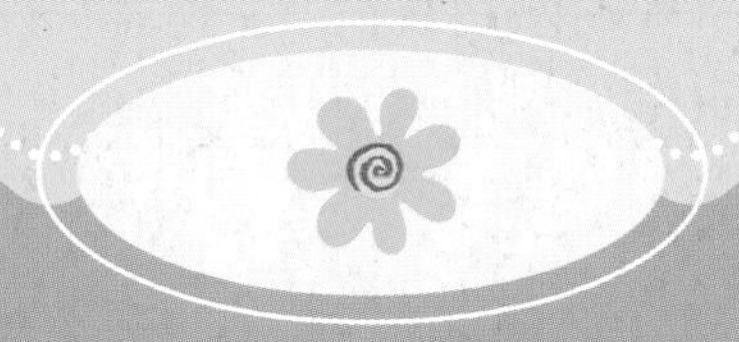

For shoulder length hair or longer.

The perfect look to show off your curl while containing the curl. Inspired by the Victorian era, the “Victorian” gives off a feeling of sweetness.

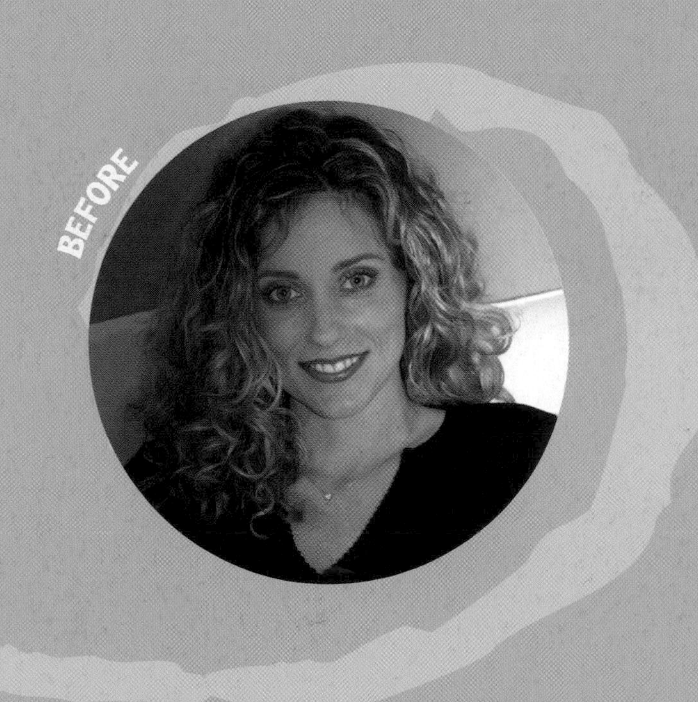

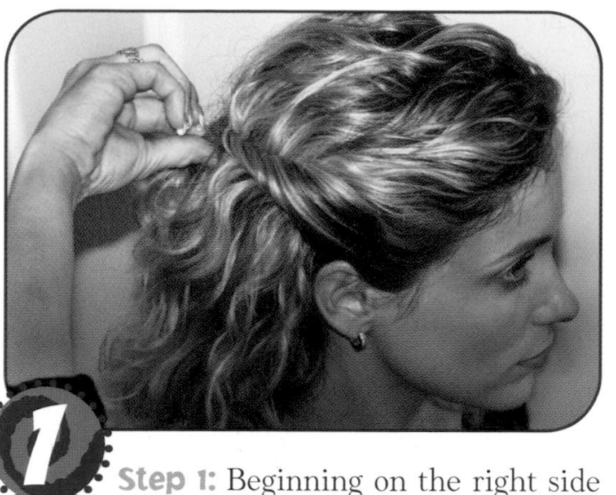

Step 1: Beginning on the right side of your head, section a two-inch by one-inch portions of hair along the hairline. Pull hair back and twist the section, pulling twisted hair to the back and center of the head. The twist should remain on the surface of the unused hair. **Note:** When pulling hair back, make sure you are just taking the hair along the hair line, leaving the majority of your hair down.

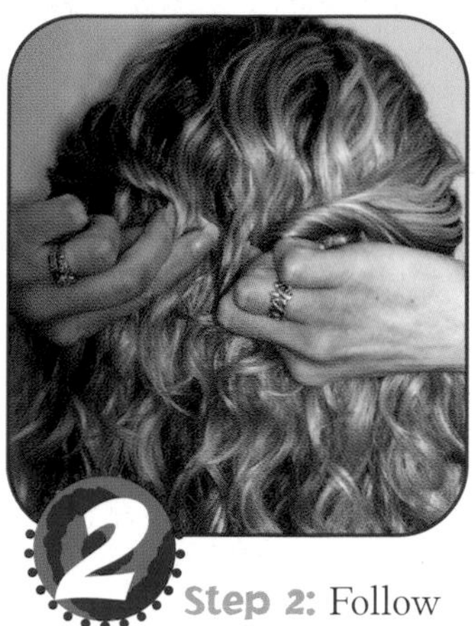

Step 2: Follow the direction in step one for the left side of the head. The twists should meet in the back at the center of your head.

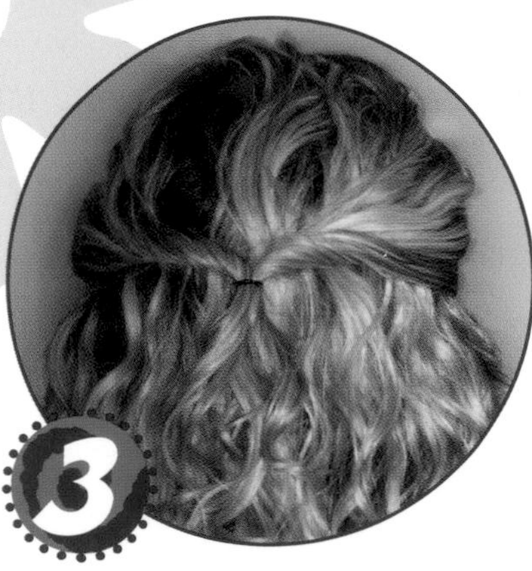

Step 3: Secure the twists with covered elastic.

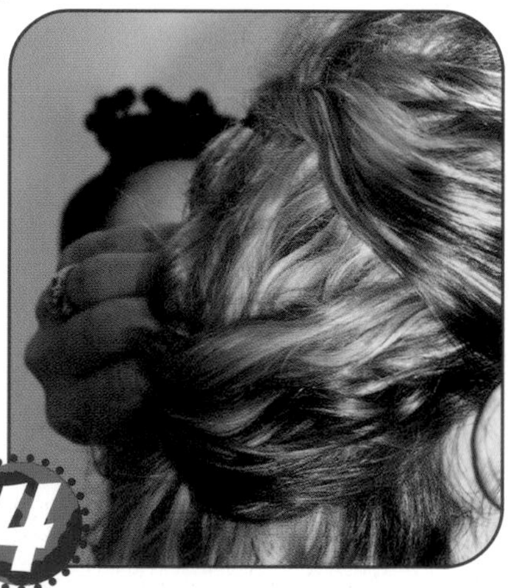

Step 4: Section a one-inch deep by two-inch long portions of hair from the right side of your head just behind the ear and twist to the back as noted in Step 1. Do the same for the left side of the head.

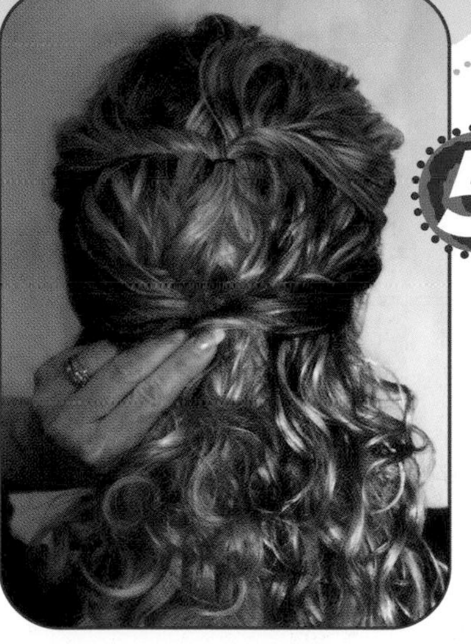

Step 5: Gather the second twists in the middle of your head just below the first twists. Secure the second set of twists with an elastic.

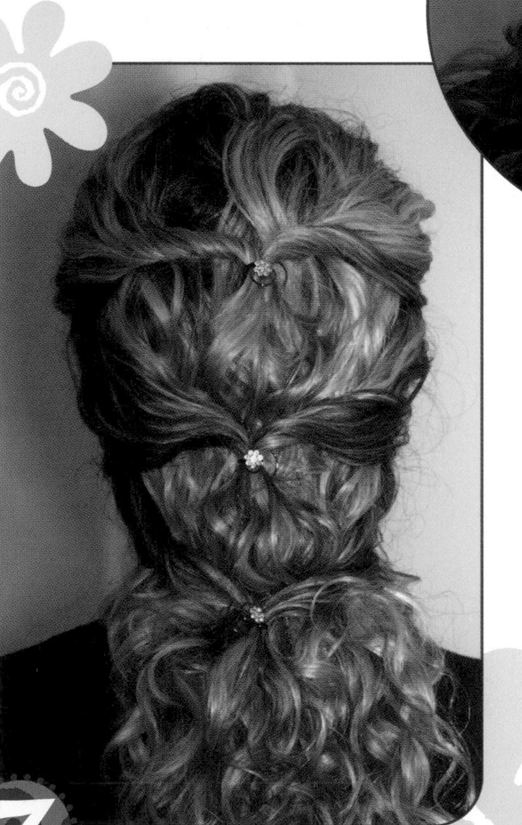

Step 6: At the nape of your neck, take the remaining hair along the right side of the hairline in a half-inch to one-inch-wide sections approximately one to two inches long and twist back.

TIP: Here we have used circular diamond accessories; ribbon of your choice is a great way to polish off the look as well.

Step 7: Repeat Step 6 on the left side, gathering the twists at the middle of the head directly below the previous twists and secure. The style is now ready for accessories.

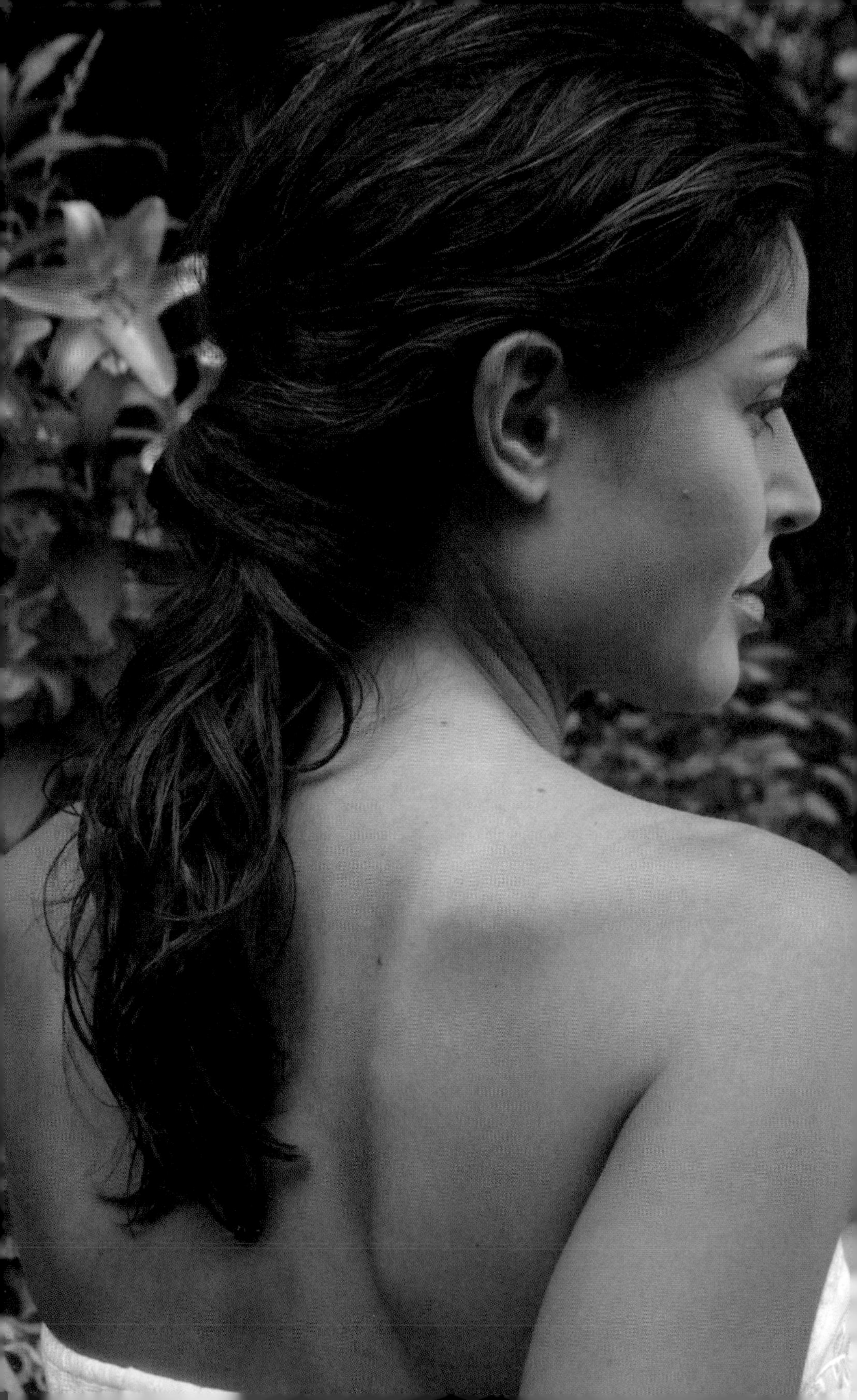

Princess

For shoulder length hair or longer.

This simple style puts an elegant twist on the otherwise boring ponytail.

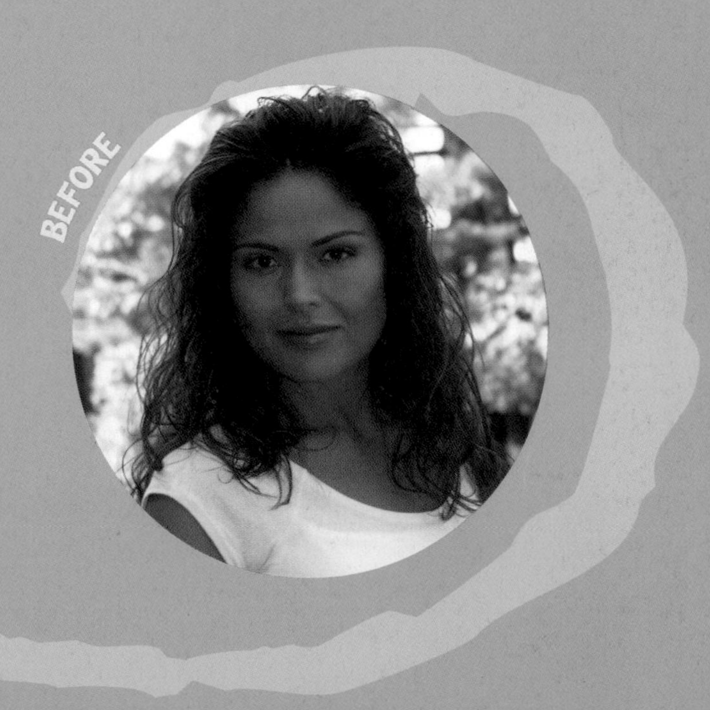

Step 1: Loosely pull hair back and into a low ponytail. Secure with covered elastic. **Note:** Use elastic similar to your hair color.

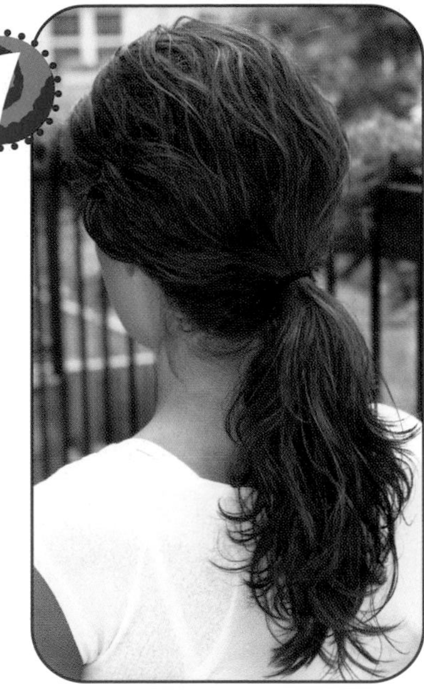

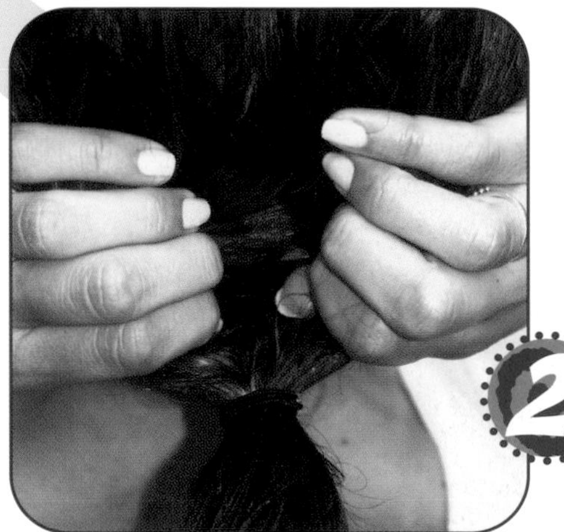

Step 2: Create a hole in the hair just above the ponytail.

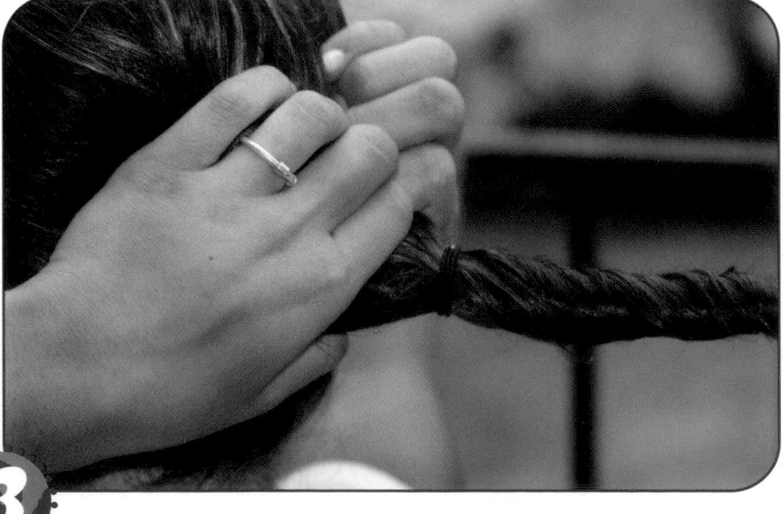

Step 3: Twist the hair in the ponytail for mobility purposes.

Step 4: Direct the twisted hair in the ponytail up, over the elastic and into the hole above the ponytail. Pull the ponytail through the hole from underneath the elastic so that the hair in the pony tail is now at the nape of the neck.

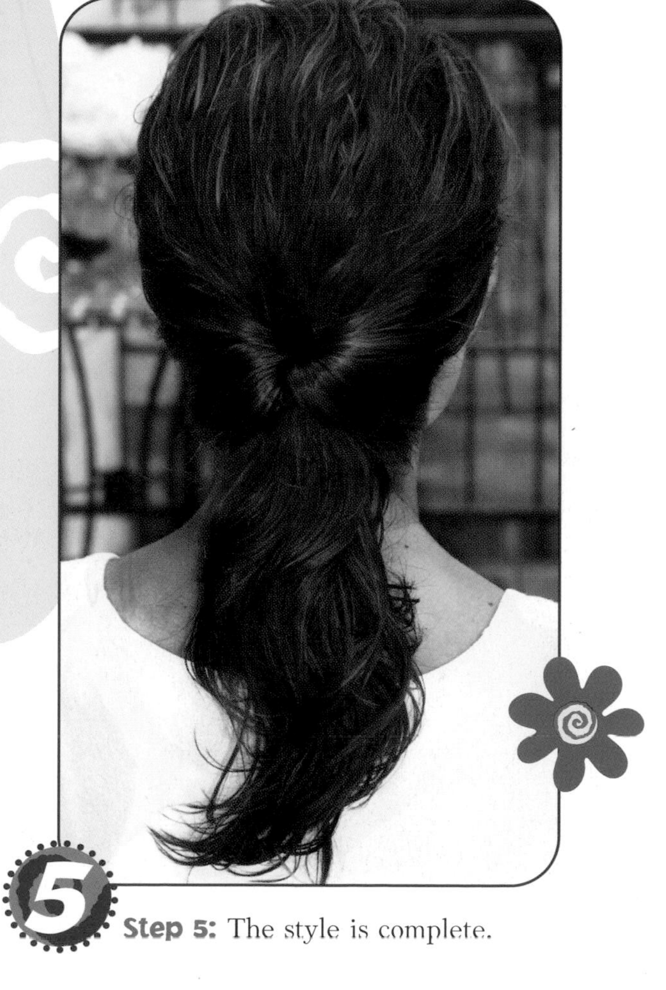

Step 5: The style is complete.

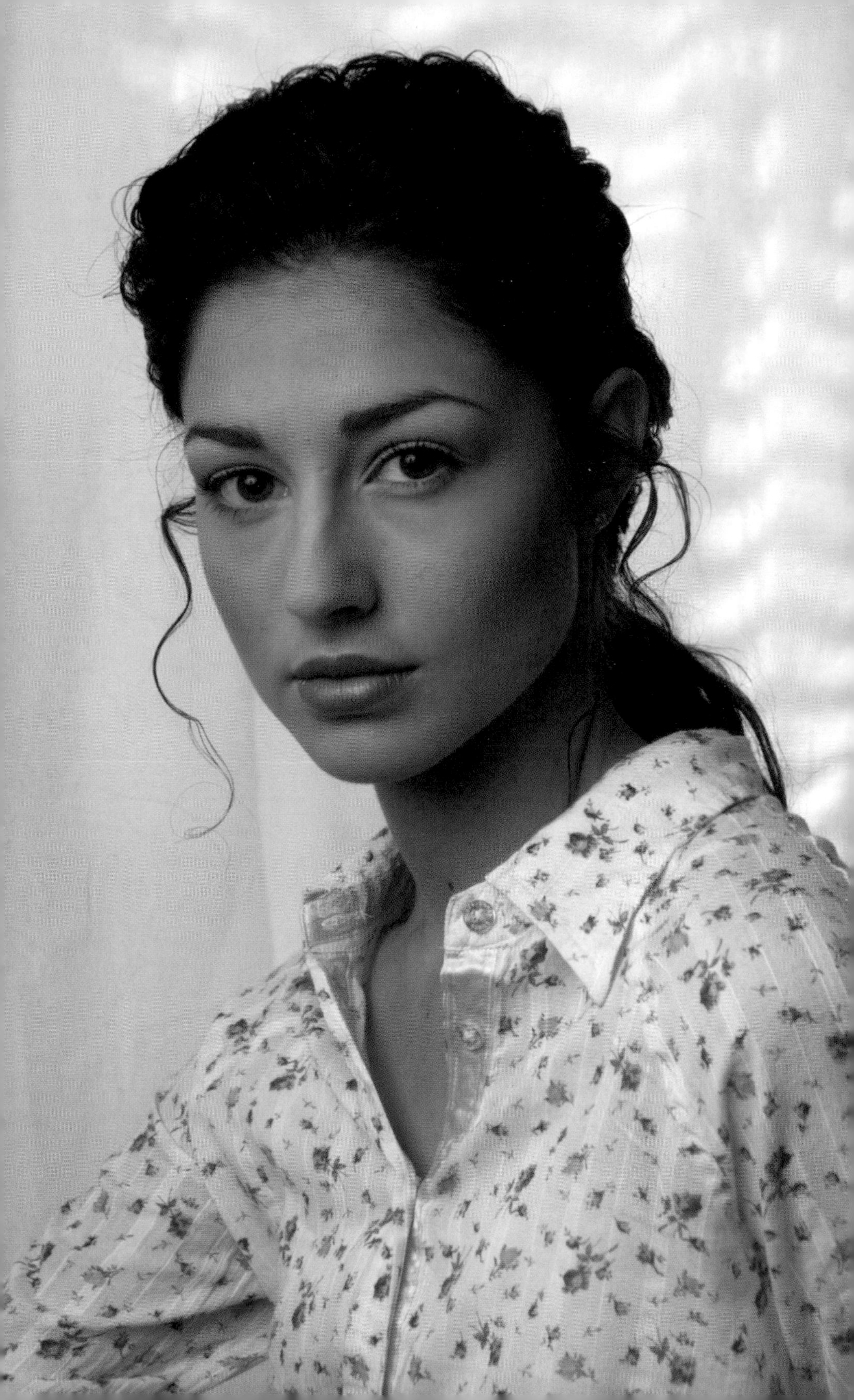

Knotty Princess

For shoulder length hair or longer.

This doubly-sweet look sings royalty, with a twist of fun!

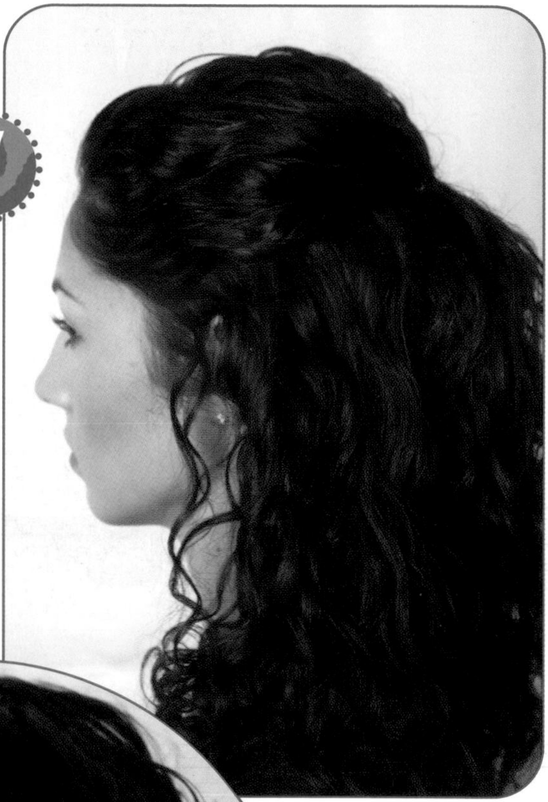

Step 1: Section hair from ear to ear around the back of head just above your occipital bone (the bump on the back of your head). Pull sectioned hair back and secure with covered elastic.

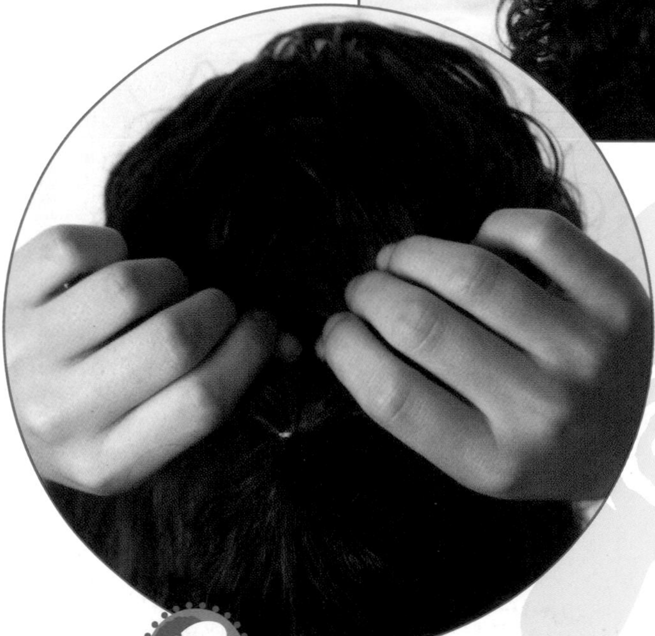

Step 2: Create a hole in the gathered hair just above the elastic.

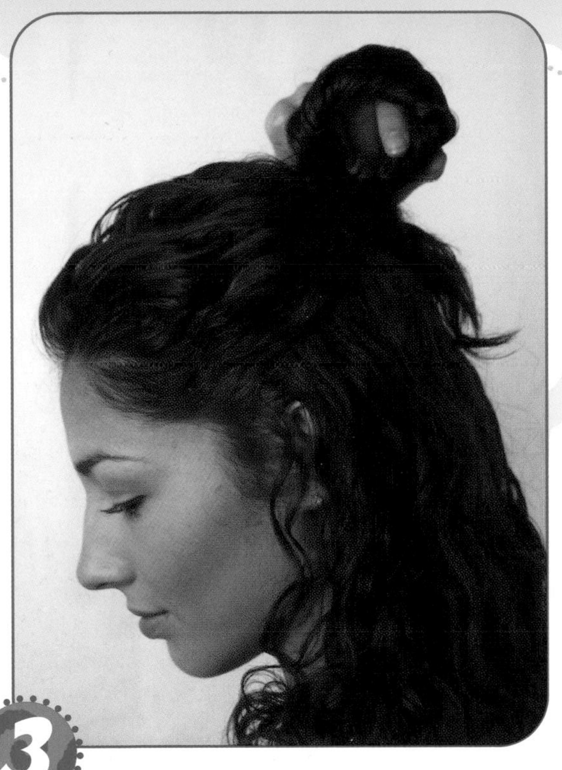

TIP:
Twisting the gathered hair into a ponytail before tucking, helps control frizz and makes it easier to pull hair through the hole.

Step 3:
Tuck the ponytail up, over the elastic and into the hole. Pull the ponytail through the hole from underneath the elastic.

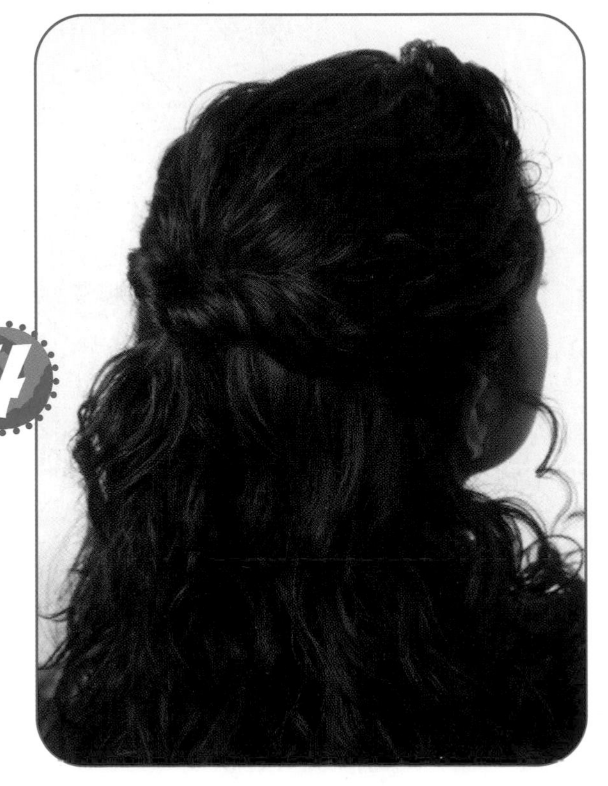

Step 4: The first princess knot is complete.

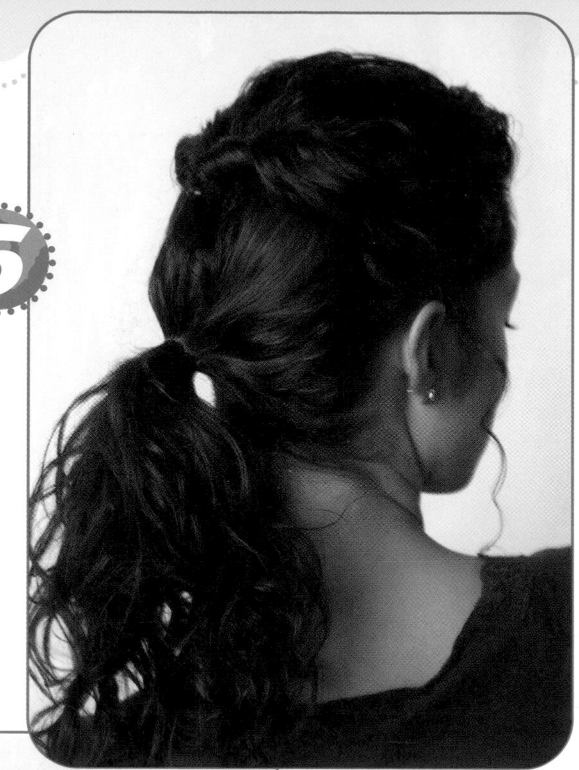

Step 5: Gather remaining hair and pull in a low ponytail at the nape of your neck. Secure ponytail with elastic.

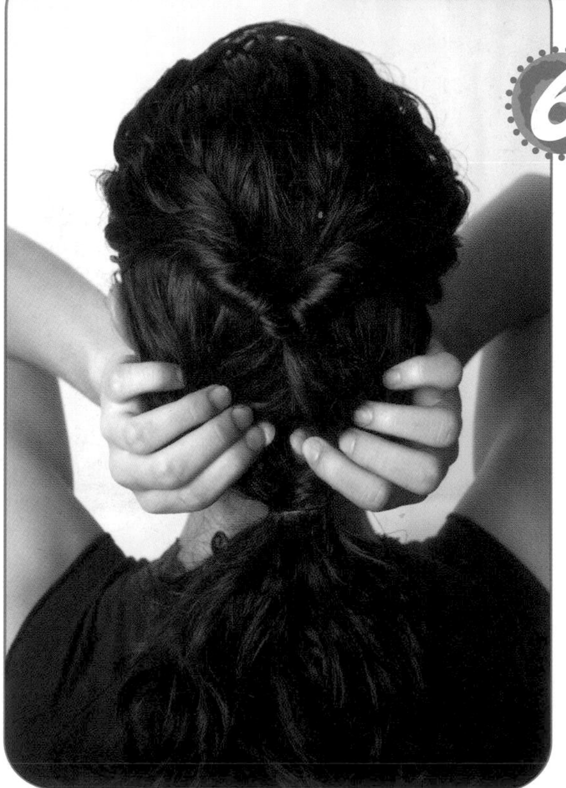

Step 6: Create a hole in the gathered hair just above the lower ponytail. Tuck hair over the top and into the hole. Pull hair through the hole from underneath the ponytail.

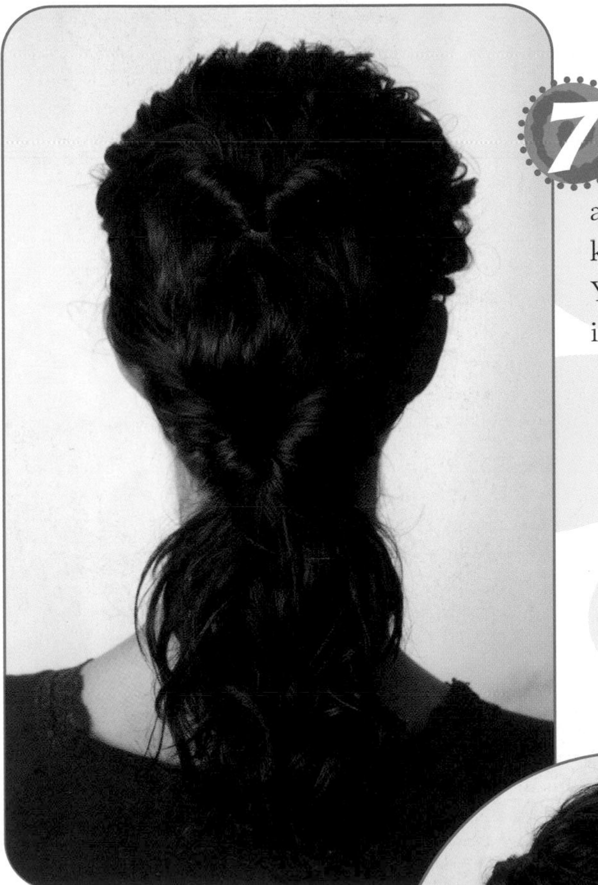

Step 7: Second and final princess knot is complete. Your knotty princess is ready to play!

TIP:
For another look, you can simply tuck all the hair hanging out up, as seen here.

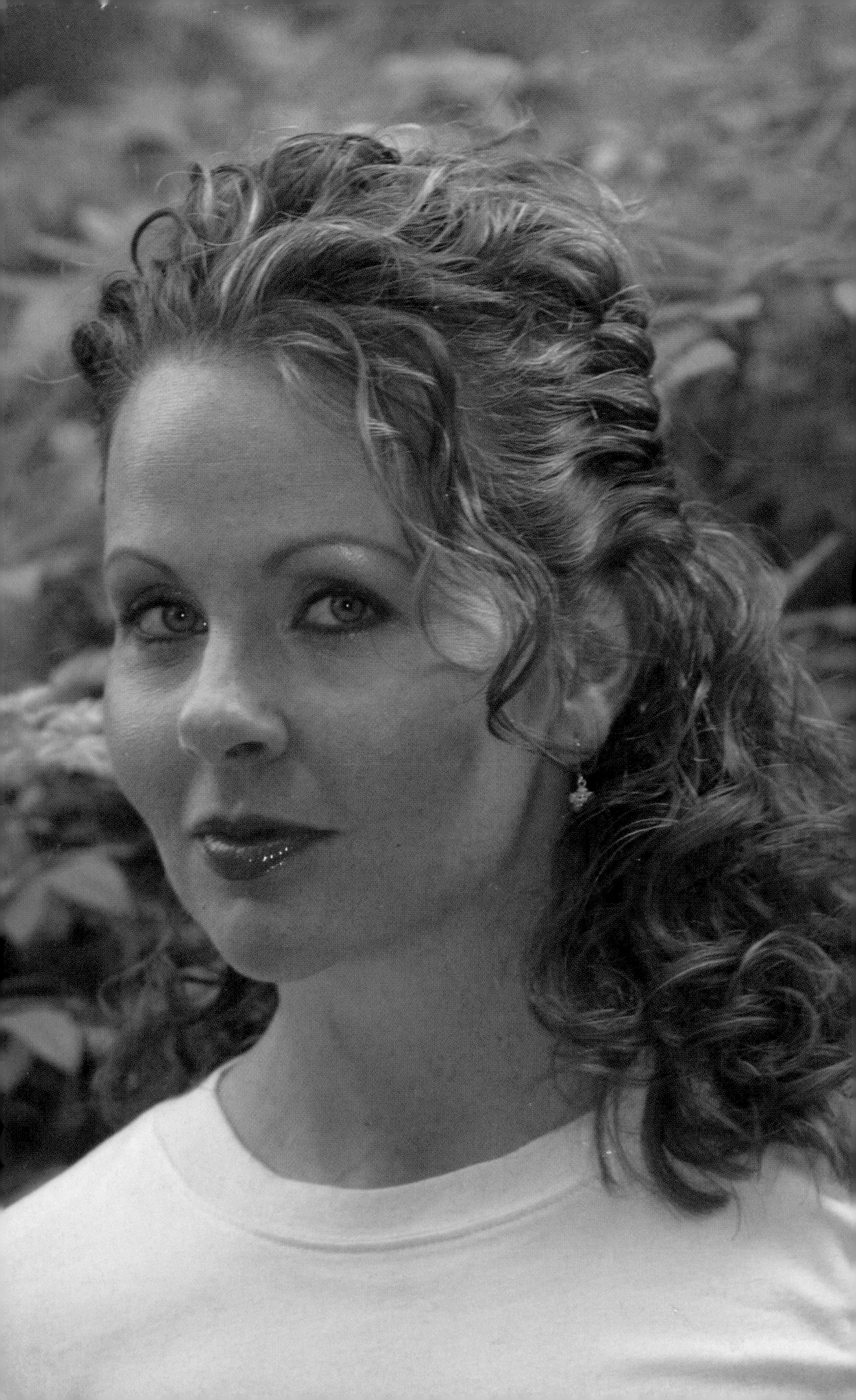

Frenchy

**For chin length hair or longer.
Layered hair is suitable**

This is fun for all medium to long hair lengths. Each length creates its own unique cascade of curls.

Step 1: Part hair on the top of your head in a manner that you favor for the finished look.

Step 2: Separate the top section of your hair from the bottom, parting hair from ear to ear. Gather the upper portion of hair and pull the section of hair to the back and center of your head.

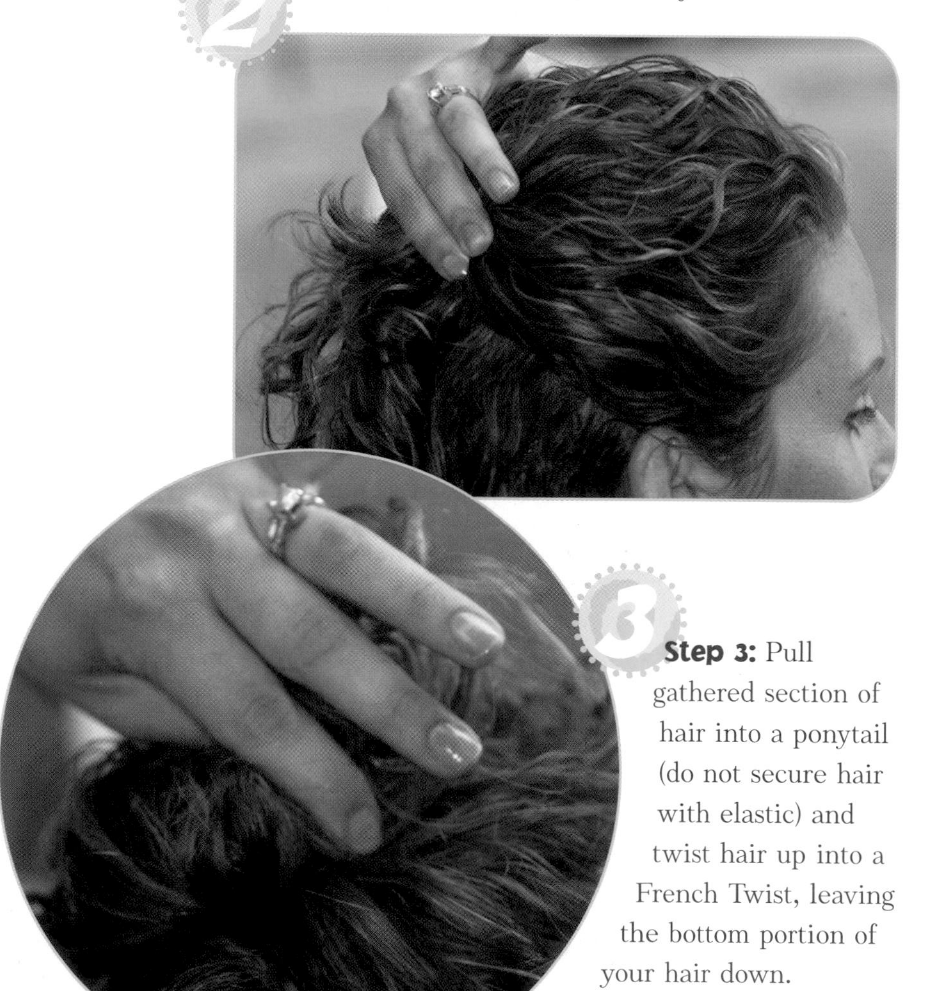

Step 3: Pull gathered section of hair into a ponytail (do not secure hair with elastic) and twist hair up into a French Twist, leaving the bottom portion of your hair down.

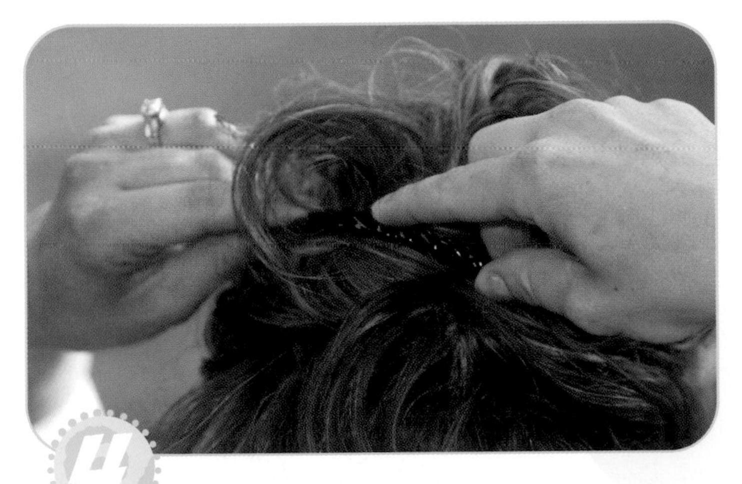

Step 4: Secure the twist with a large barrette. If twist is too thick for a barrette, use two-inch bobby pins to secure the twist.

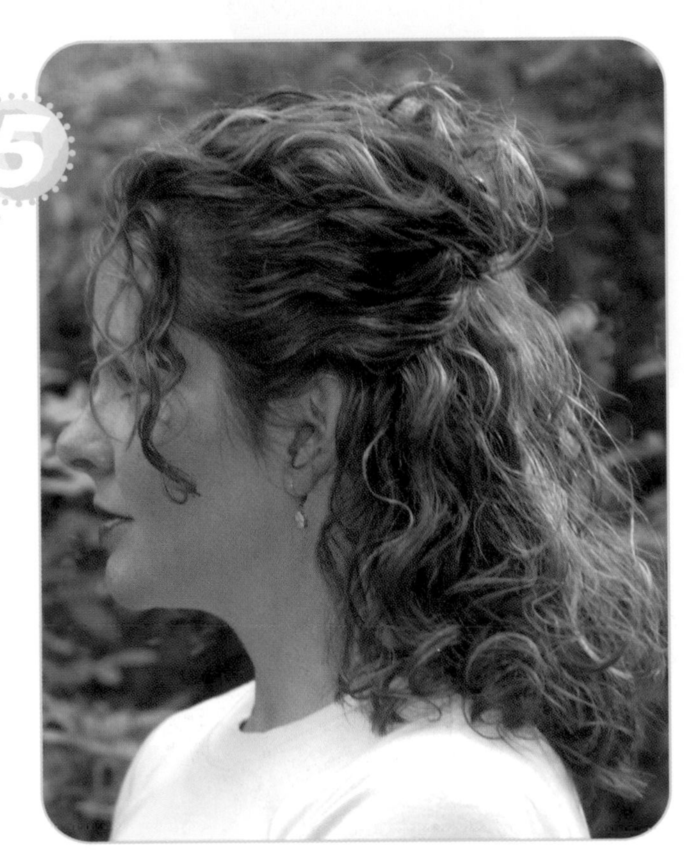

Step 5: Fluff the ends of the twist that are sprouting up and cascading down over the twist. Add accessories to your taste.

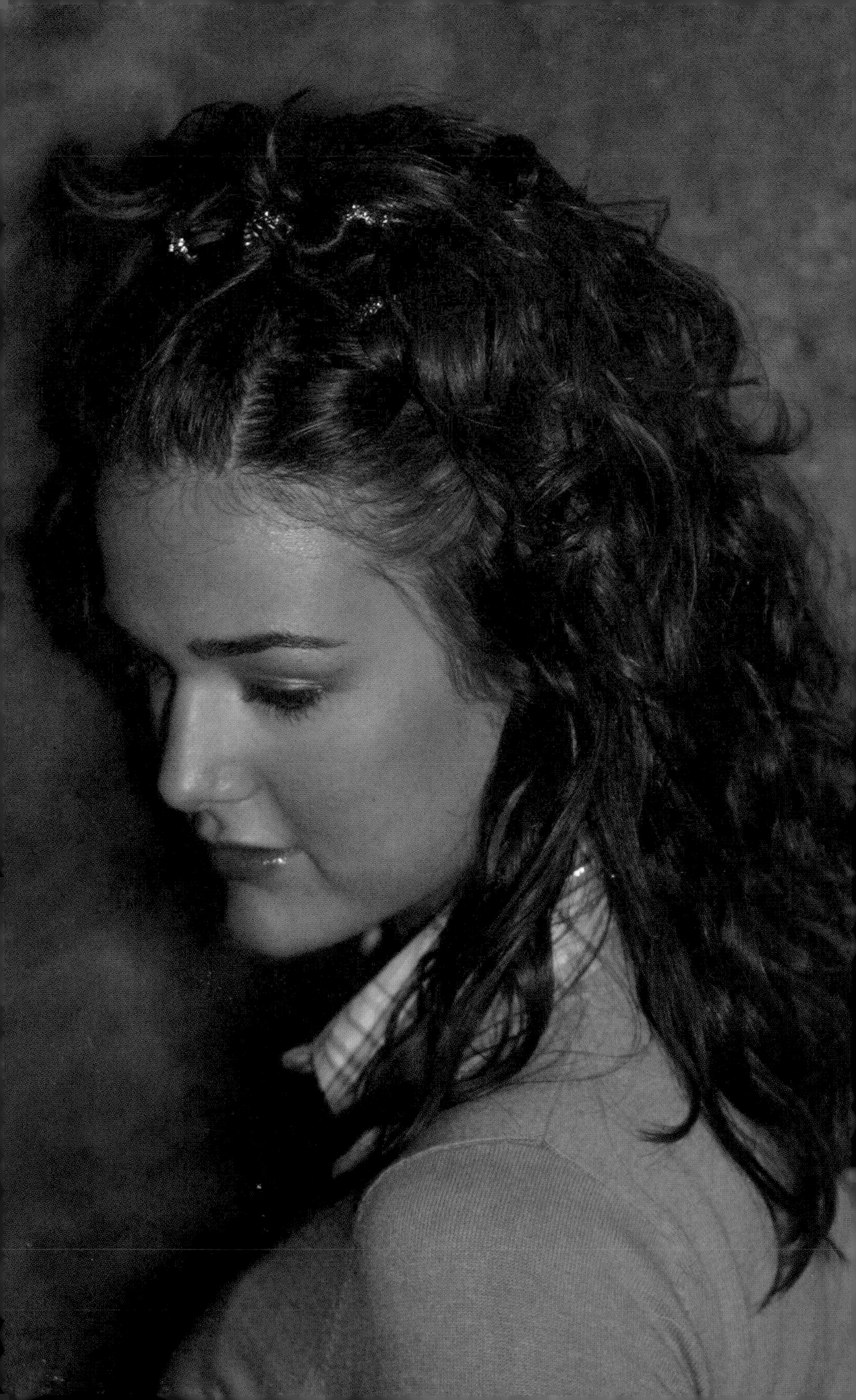

Knotty Knots

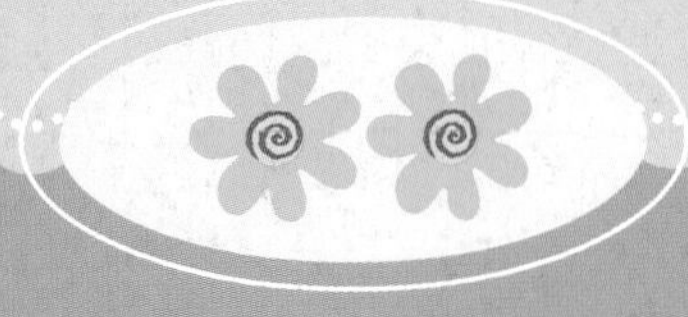

For chin length hair or longer.
Longer layers work well
with this style

Perfectly playful. This is a great look to spice up any outfit.

Step 1: Gather a one-half-inch by one-half-inch section of hair at the crown of the head.

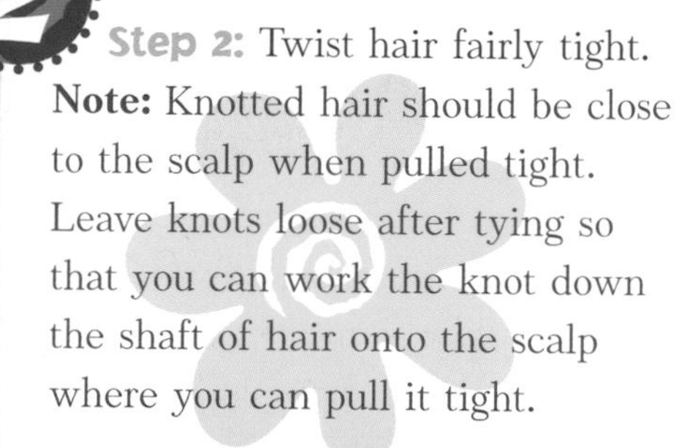

Step 2: Twist hair fairly tight. **Note:** Knotted hair should be close to the scalp when pulled tight. Leave knots loose after tying so that you can work the knot down the shaft of hair onto the scalp where you can pull it tight.

Step 3: Tie a knot with the twisted hair as you would a rope and secure with bobby pins. **Note:** When applying a bobby pin to the knotted hair, straddle the legs of the pin over a portion of the knotted hair. Press the pin downward onto the scalp and then push the pin forward through the bottom of the knot.

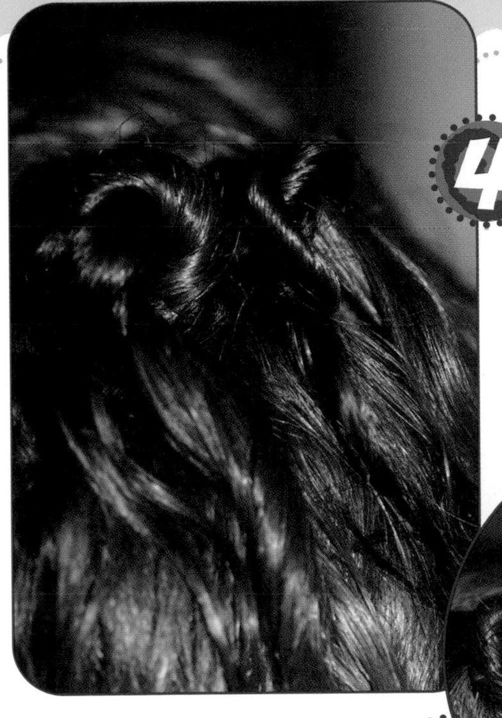

4

Step 4: Gather a second section of hair to the right of the first knot. Twist hair, tie into a knot and secure with bobby pins.

5

Step 5: Twist and tie a third knot to the left of the first knot. You should have three knots positioned across the crown of your head.

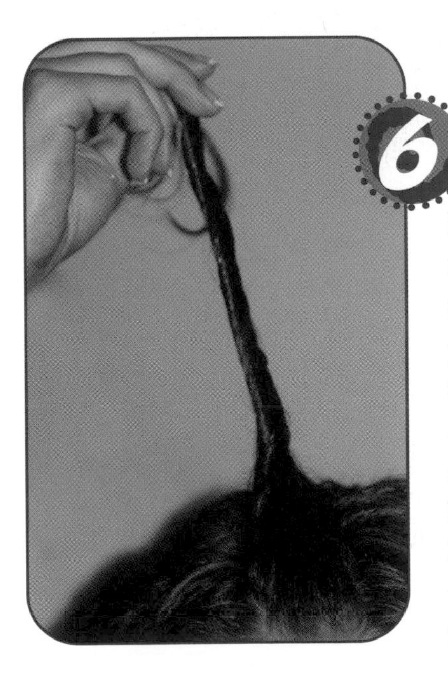

6

Step 6: Now begin with the hair along the hairline. Gather a section of hair at the top and center of your forehead. The portion of hair should be about one inch wide and two to four inches deep towards your existing knots at the crown of the head. Twist sectioned hair toward the existing knots. Be sure to twist the hair with moderate tension compensate for the knotted hair loosening.

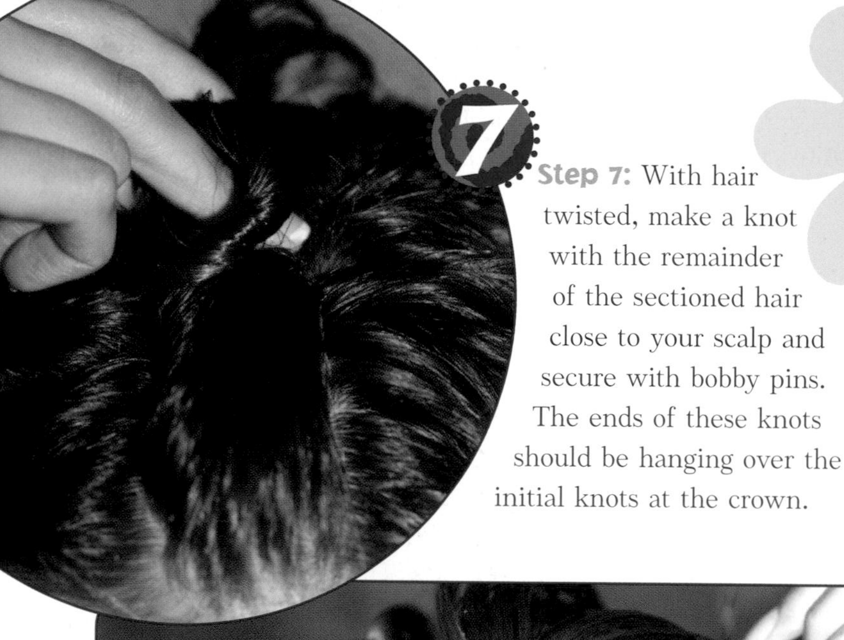

Step 7: With hair twisted, make a knot with the remainder of the sectioned hair close to your scalp and secure with bobby pins. The ends of these knots should be hanging over the initial knots at the crown.

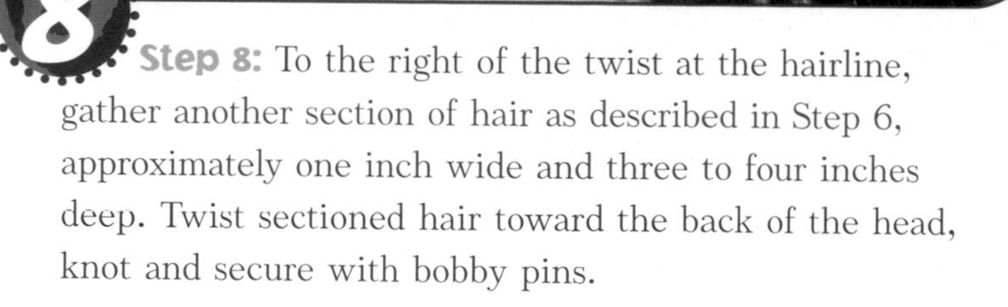

Step 8: To the right of the twist at the hairline, gather another section of hair as described in Step 6, approximately one inch wide and three to four inches deep. Twist sectioned hair toward the back of the head, knot and secure with bobby pins.

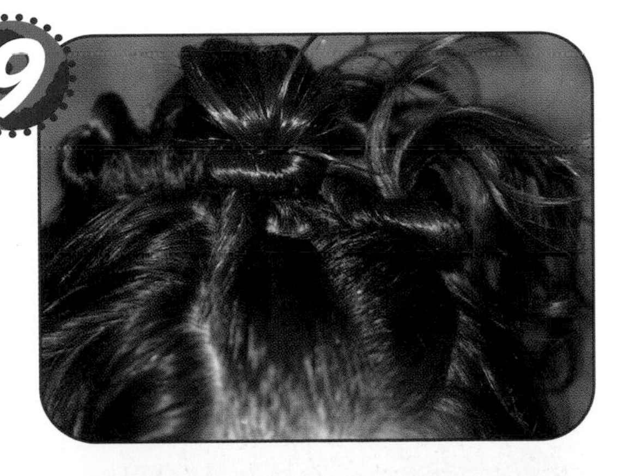

Step 9: Create a third hairline twist to the left of the center twist following the directions in Step 9. Depending on your hairline, you can add two more with a total of five twist back knots.

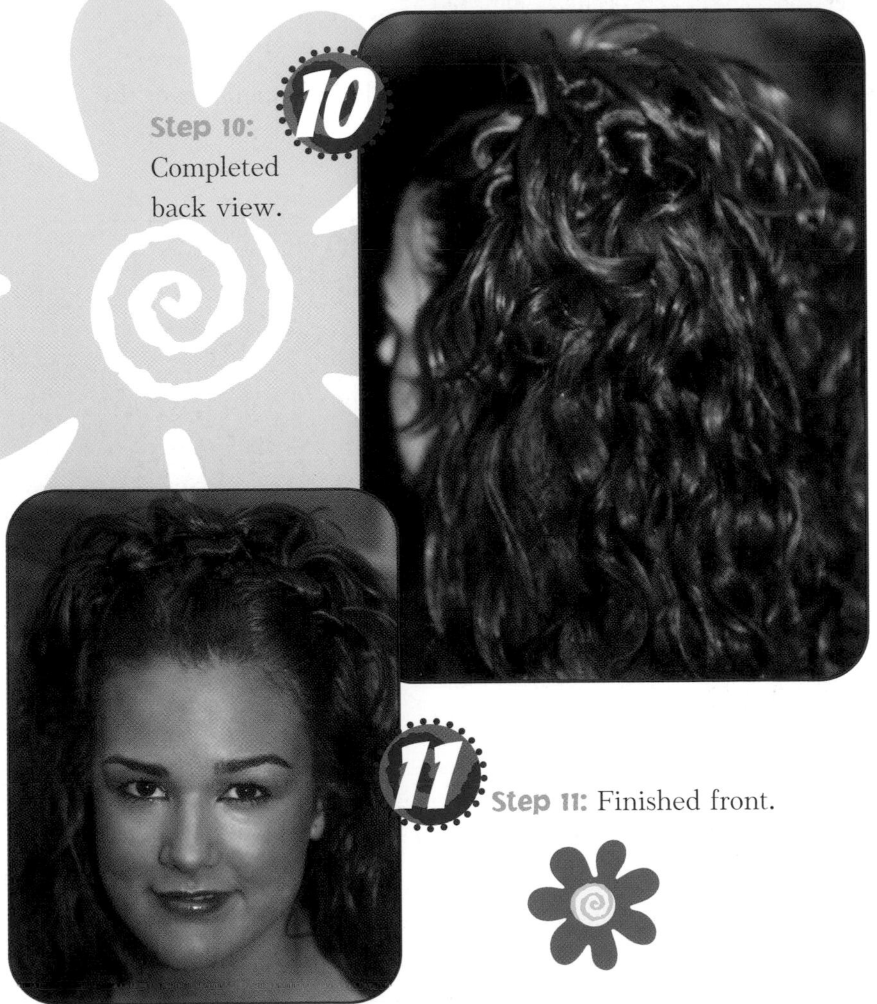

Step 10: Completed back view.

Step 11: Finished front.

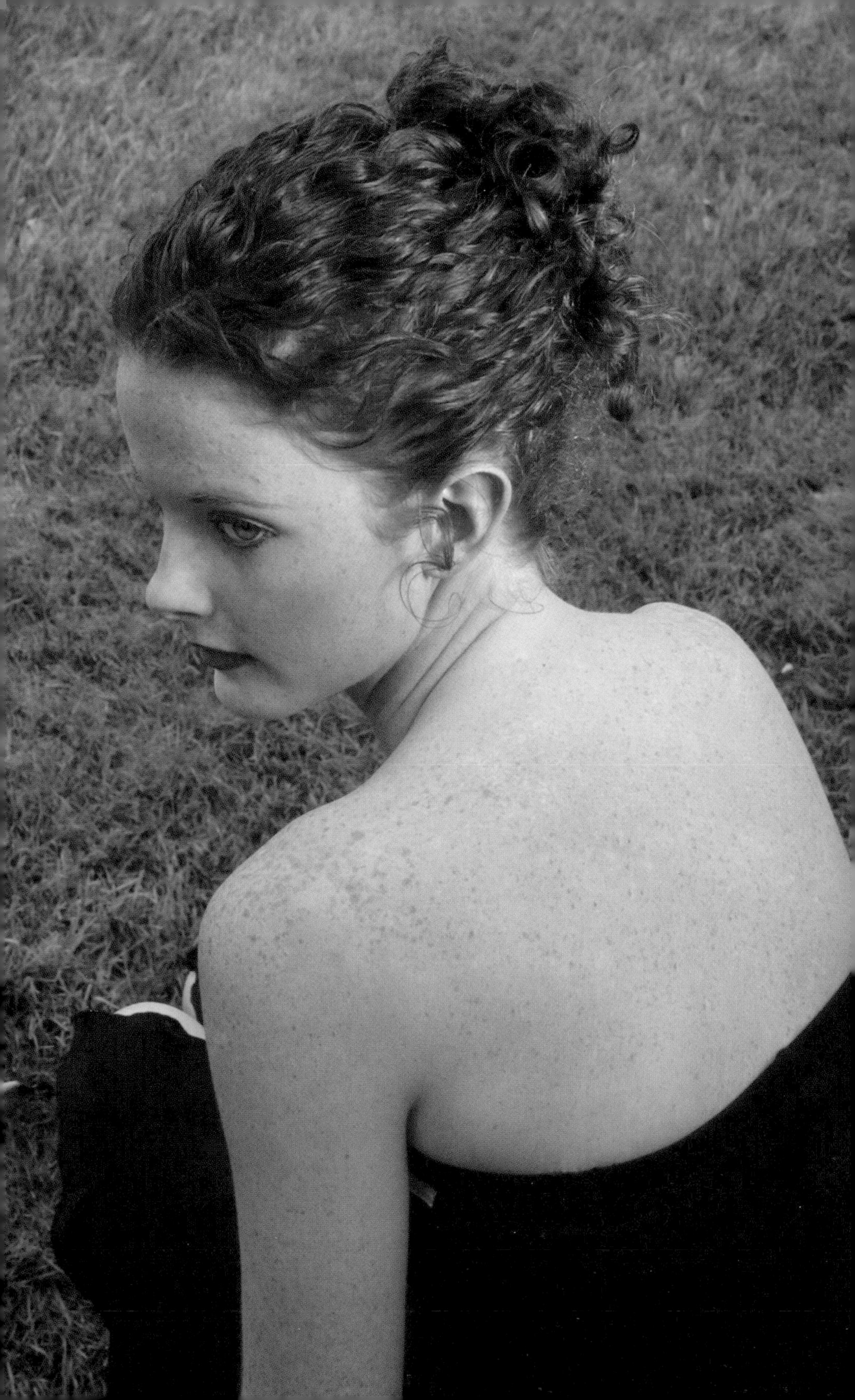

Twistd'doodle

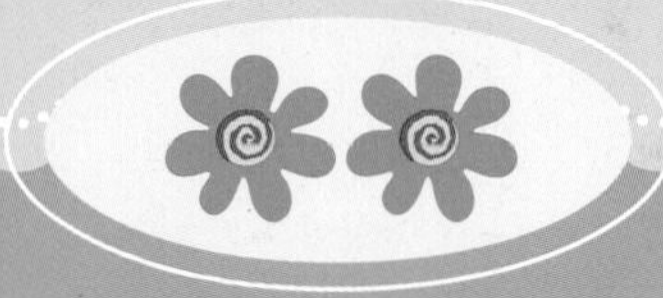

For shoulder length hair or longer.

Sleek and sophisticated. Three buns gingerly placed about the back of your head create interest and intrigue.

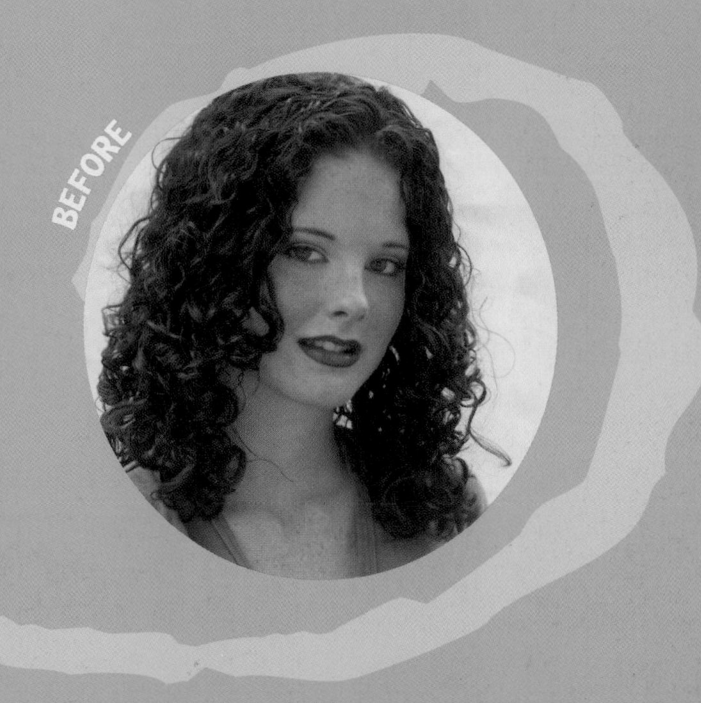

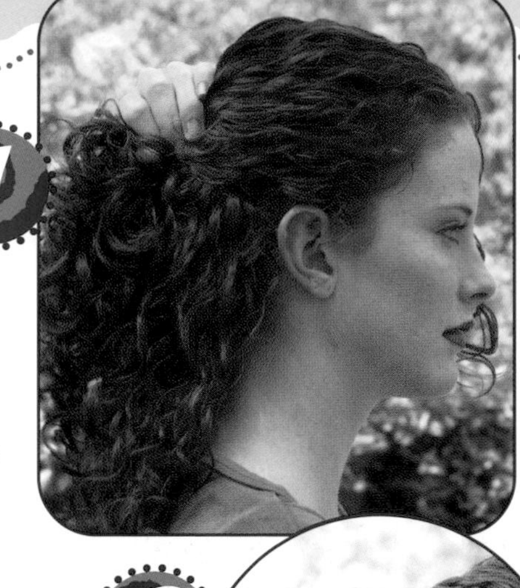

Step 1: Section the top and front of your hair from the hairline to the crown and from ear to ear on the sides. Gather hair. Pull a few small curls from the gathered hair to create fringe around the face.

Step 2: Twist gathered hair counterclockwise.

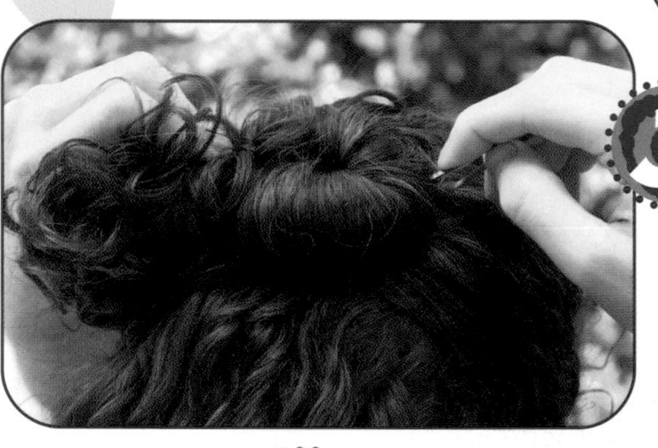

Step 3: Continue to twist hair into a bun, leaving the ends out. Place bun just below or at the crown of your head and secure.

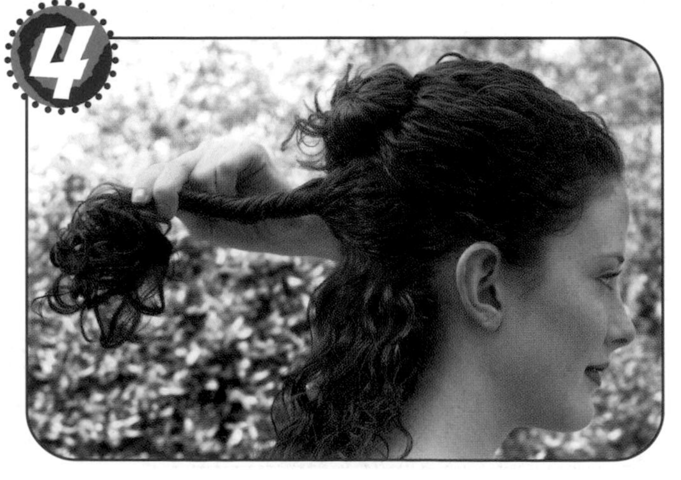

Step 4: Divide remaining loose hair to create a top section and a bottom section. Gather top section of hair and twist clockwise into a second bun.

Step 5: When the second bun is complete, the ends should be sticking out the opposite side from the bun above. Secure this bun just off center to the bun above.

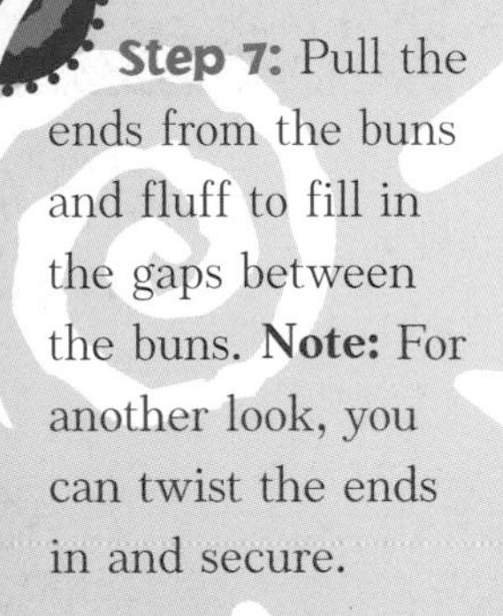

Step 6: Twist remaining hair counterclockwise up. Create a bun and place directly under the first bun. Secure with a bobby pin.

Step 7: Pull the ends from the buns and fluff to fill in the gaps between the buns. **Note:** For another look, you can twist the ends in and secure.

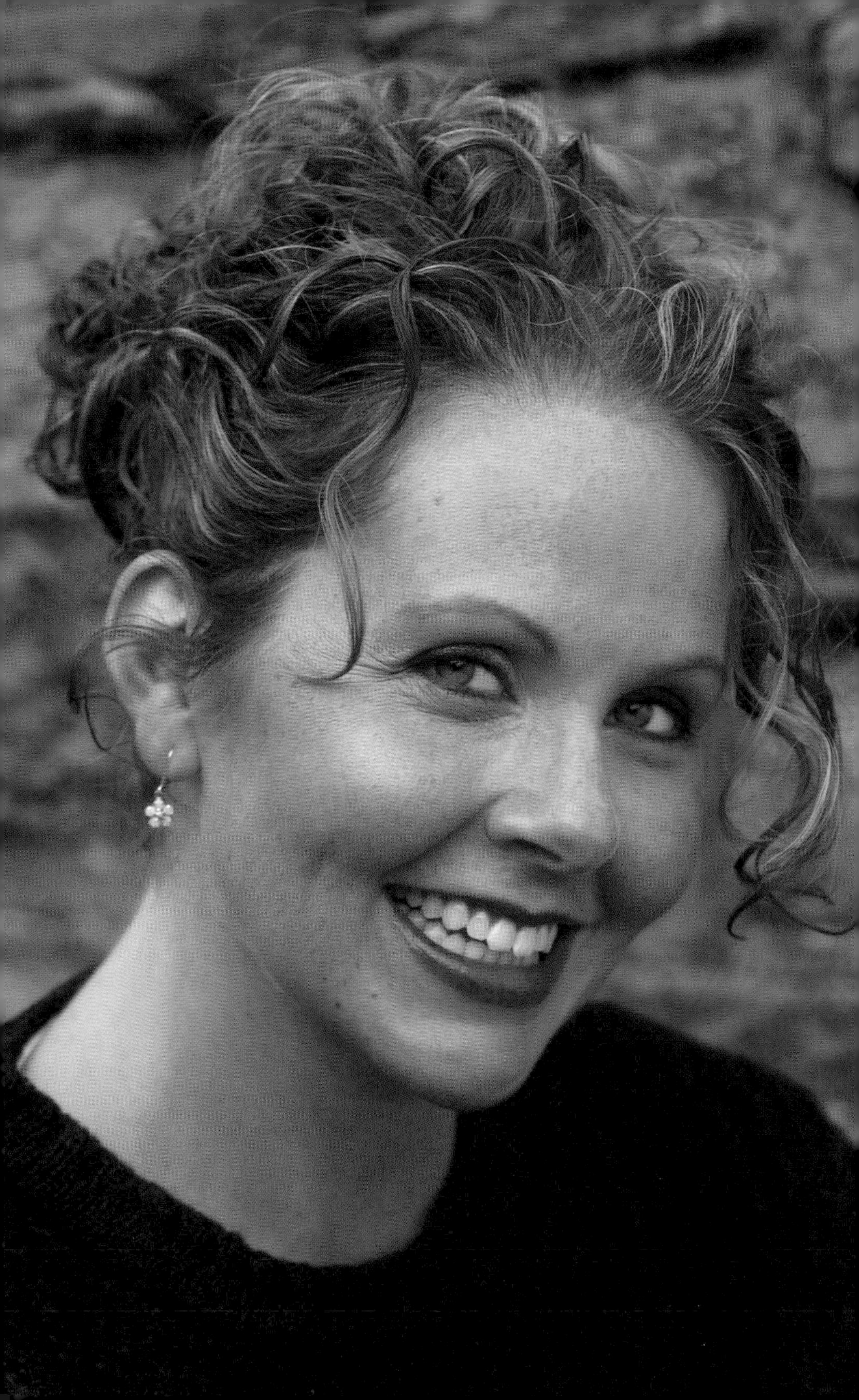

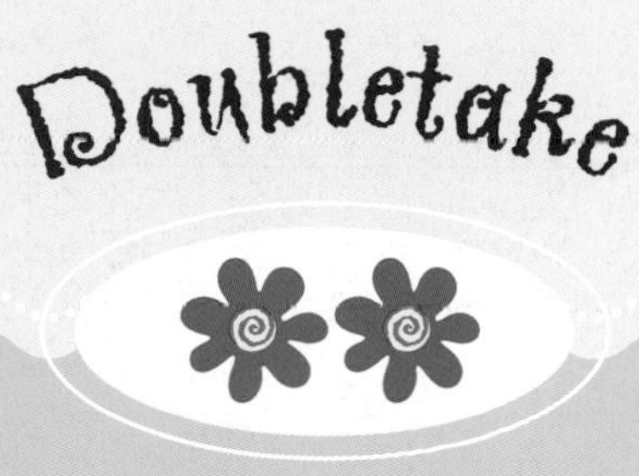

For shoulder length hair or longer.

Inspired by the traditional French twist, this look adds interest to your tresses by creating fullness at the top of the head and down the back, making for a flattering look from all angles.

Step 1: Divide hair from ear to ear, using your occipital bone (this is the bump on the back of your head) as a guide. Gather the hair above the bone. Pull hair back.

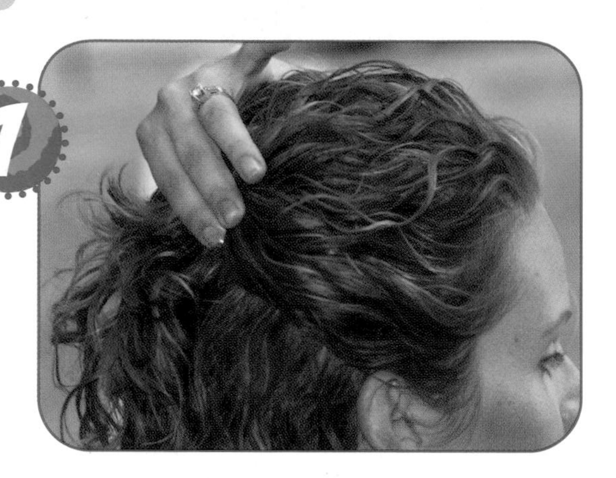

Step 2: Simply take the gathered hair and twist it up as you would for French twist.

Step 3: Secure with a large barrette. Two-inch bobby pins may be used to secure twist as well.

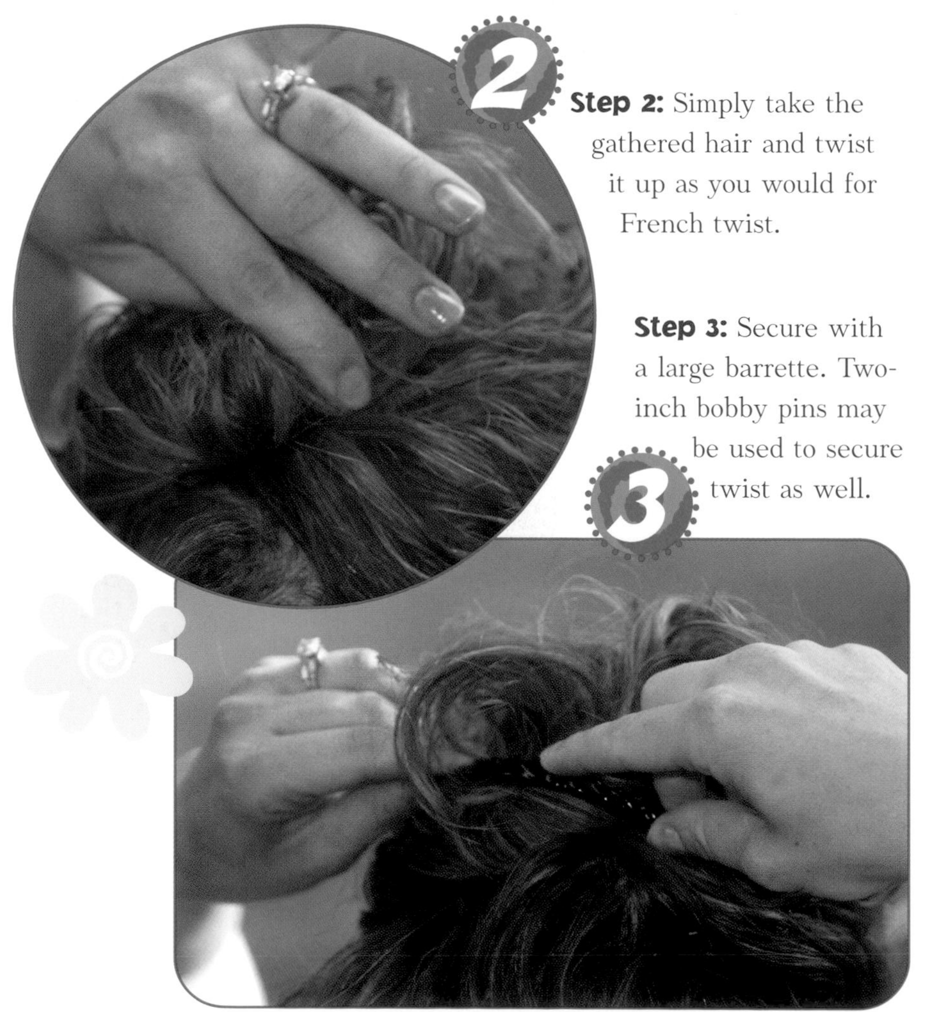

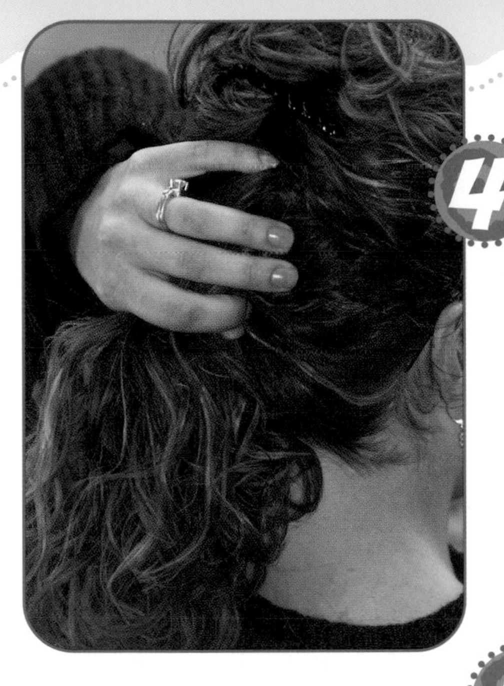

Step 4: Take the bottom half of your hair and pull into a ponytail.

Step 5: Twist the bottom section of your hair in the same manner as you did the top. Make sure the twists are close together. Secure with a barrette and fluff curls for balance.

Step 6: Shown here, the two twists are close enough together that the outcome looks like one big cluster of curls and not two separate twists.

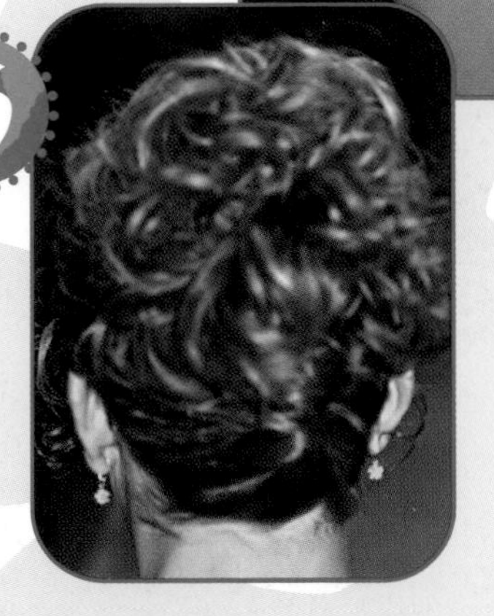

Note: If you would rather use bobby pins for this look, open the bobby pin slightly and take a little hair from the twist with one leg of the pin. With the other leg take a little hair on your head. Press the booby pin into the twist pushing it down towards the scalp and into the twist. For thick hair you may have more success with a large bobby pin.

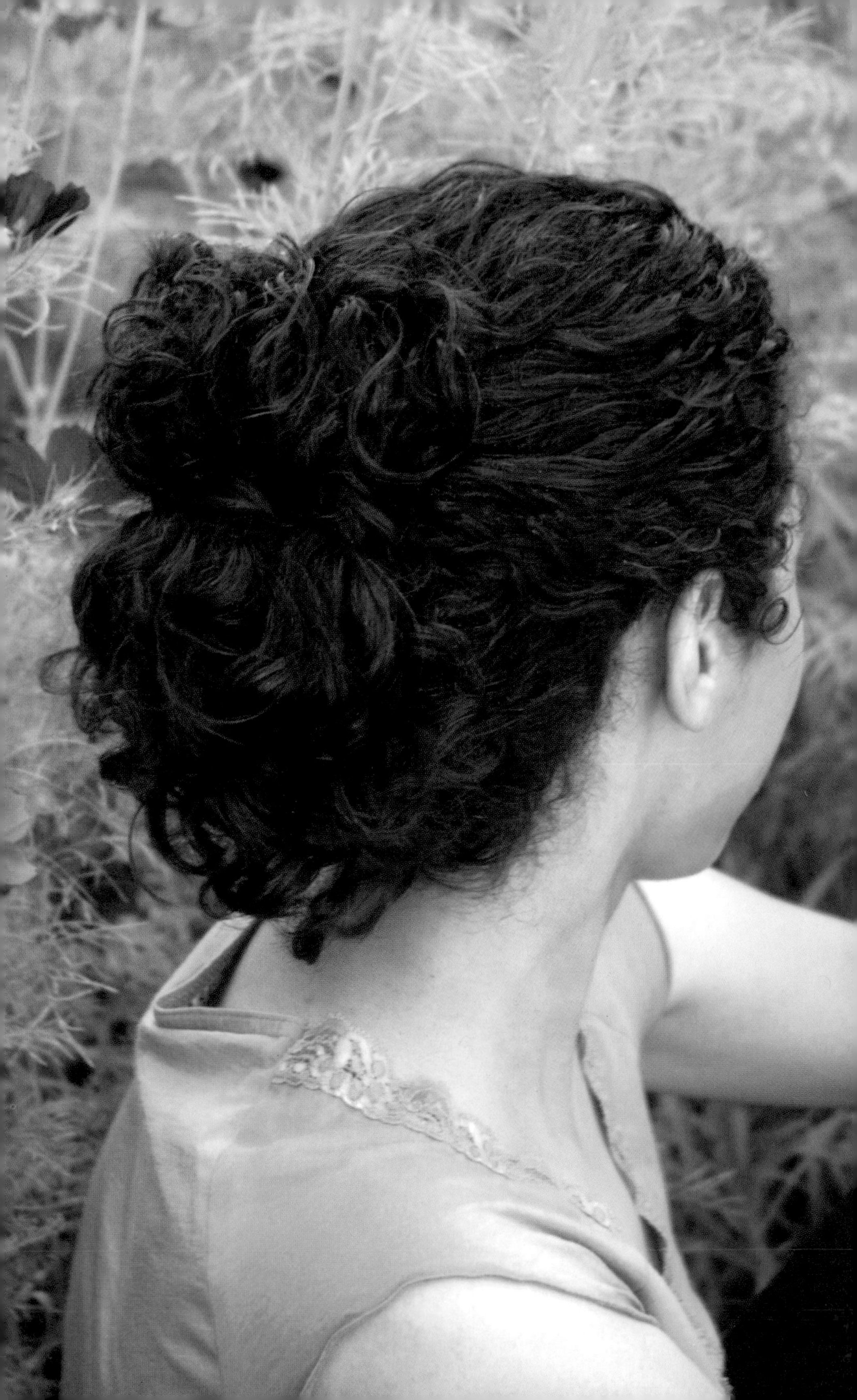

Butterfly

**For shoulder length hair.
Long layers are appropriate.**

Sensitive and sweet! This style emulates a butterfly in more ways than one. Made up of two pony tails and indicated by the flowers you'll have an easy time creating this peaceful look.

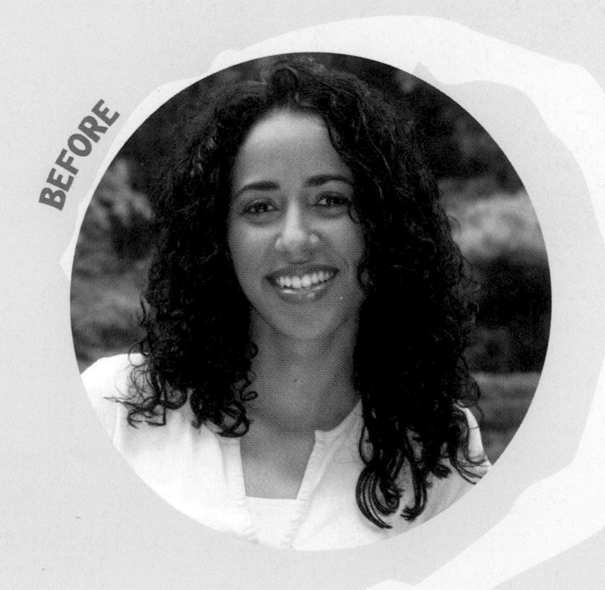

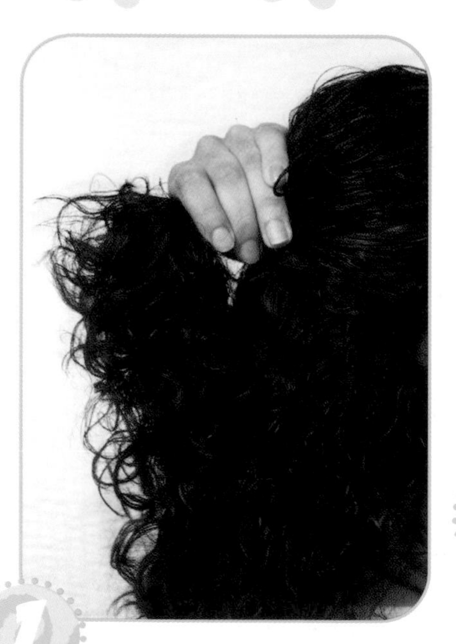

Step 1: Section the top and front of your hair from the hairline to the crown and from ear to ear on the sides. Gather hair. Pull a few small curls from the gathered hair to create fringe around the face.

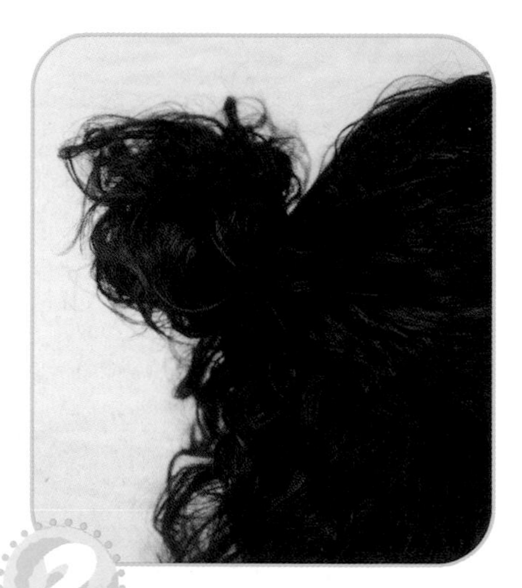

Step 2: With covered elastic, put hair into a ponytail but do not pull it all the way through. Catch the hair mid-shaft so the hair bends, creating a barrel, and the ends are left out.

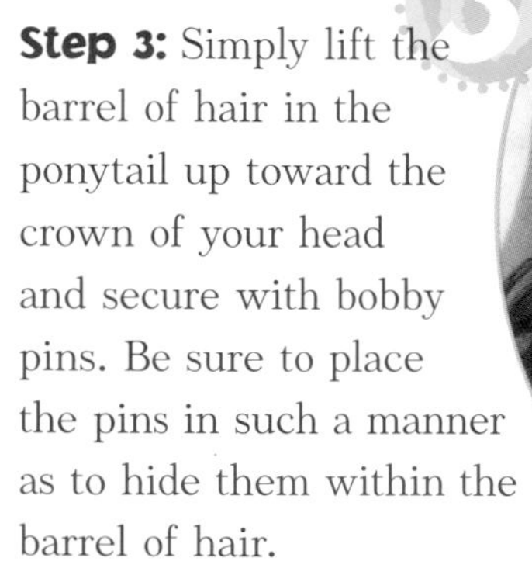

Step 3: Simply lift the barrel of hair in the ponytail up toward the crown of your head and secure with bobby pins. Be sure to place the pins in such a manner as to hide them within the barrel of hair.

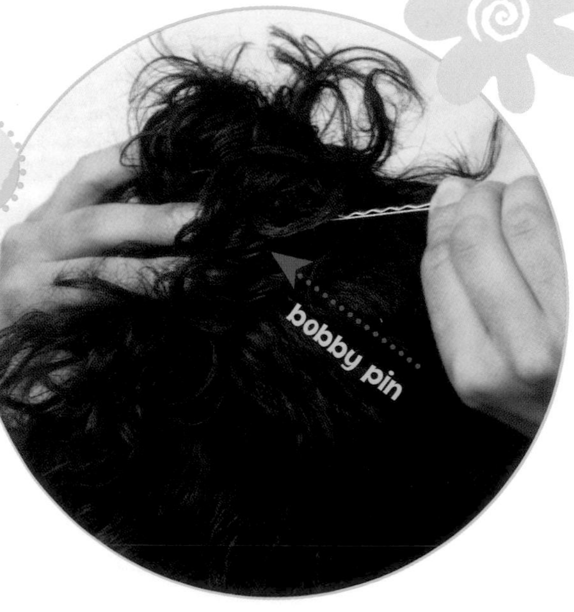

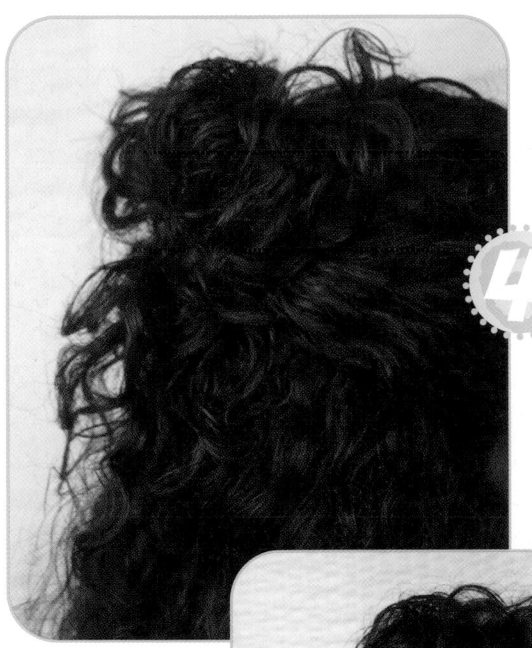

Step 4: The barrel should be lying parallel to the head in contrast to Step 2.

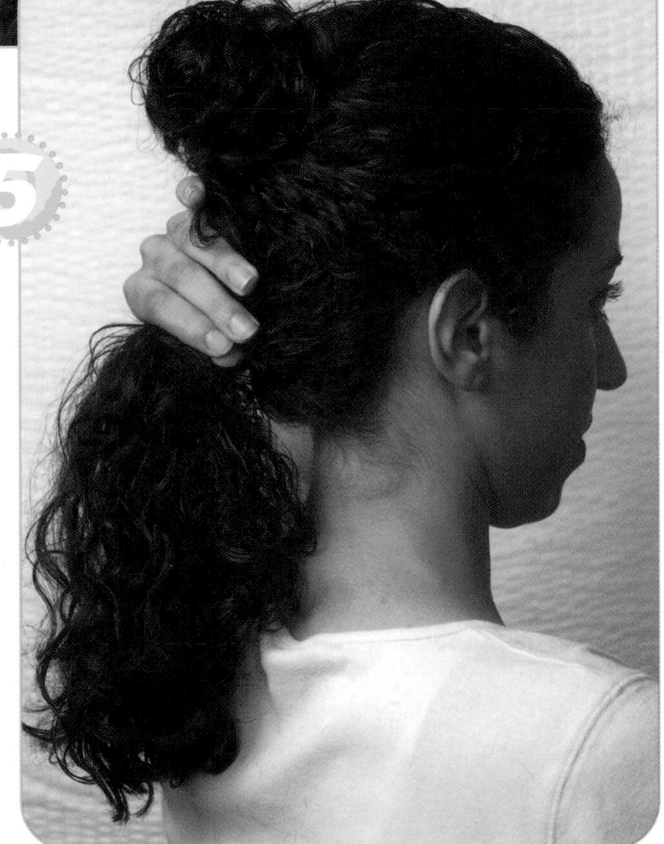

Step 5: Gather the bottom portion of hair on the head into a ponytail.

TIP—securing your bobby pin in place: At the barrel entrance, make sure you first push the bobby pin towards the scalp, then weave it through the barrel.

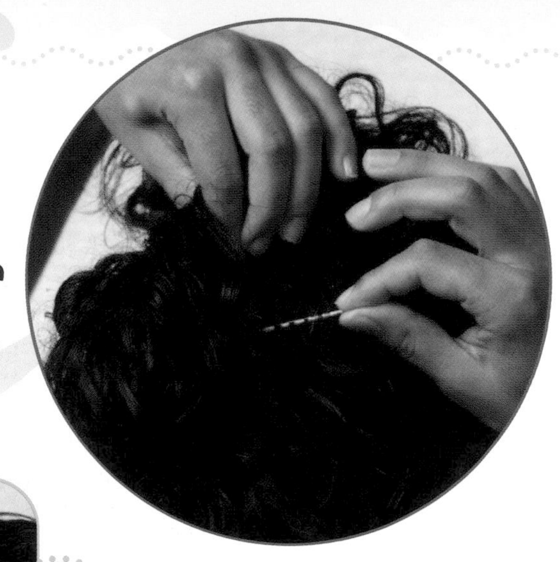

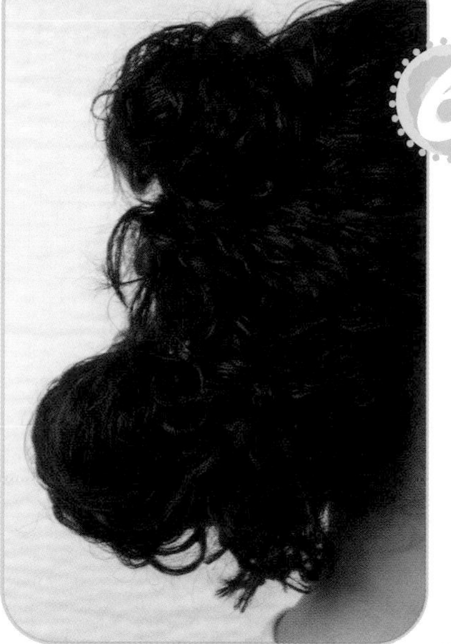

6

Step 6: Make a ponytail and do not pull it all the way through as mentioned in Step 2. Again, catch the hair mid shaft, leaving the ends out.

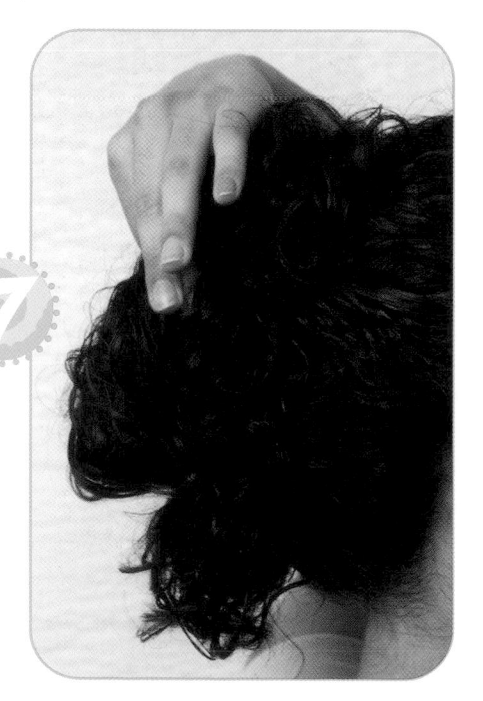

7

Step 7: Lift and pin second barrel, forming symmetry between the two knobs.

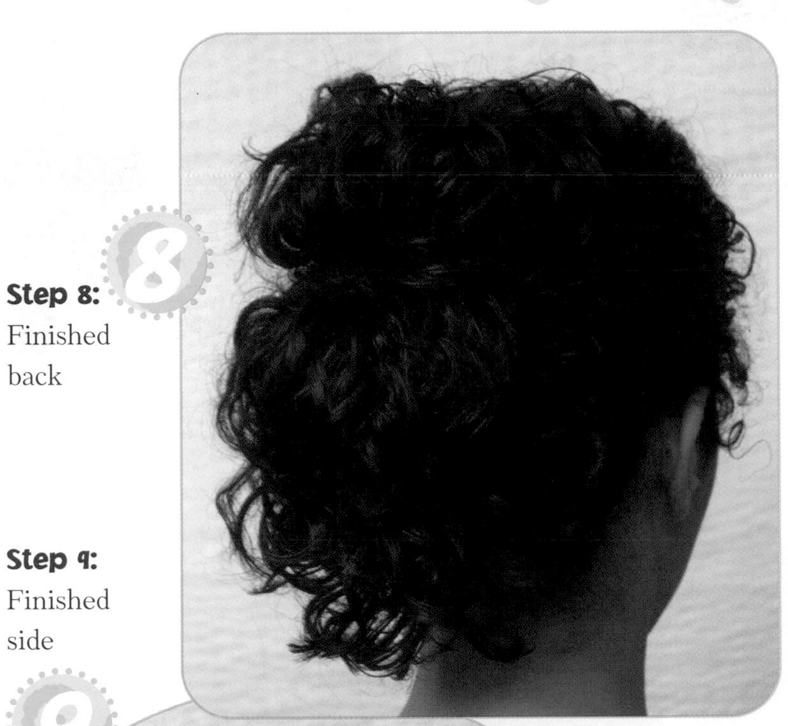

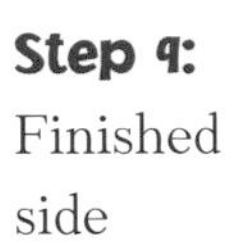

Step 8: Finished back

Step 9: Finished side

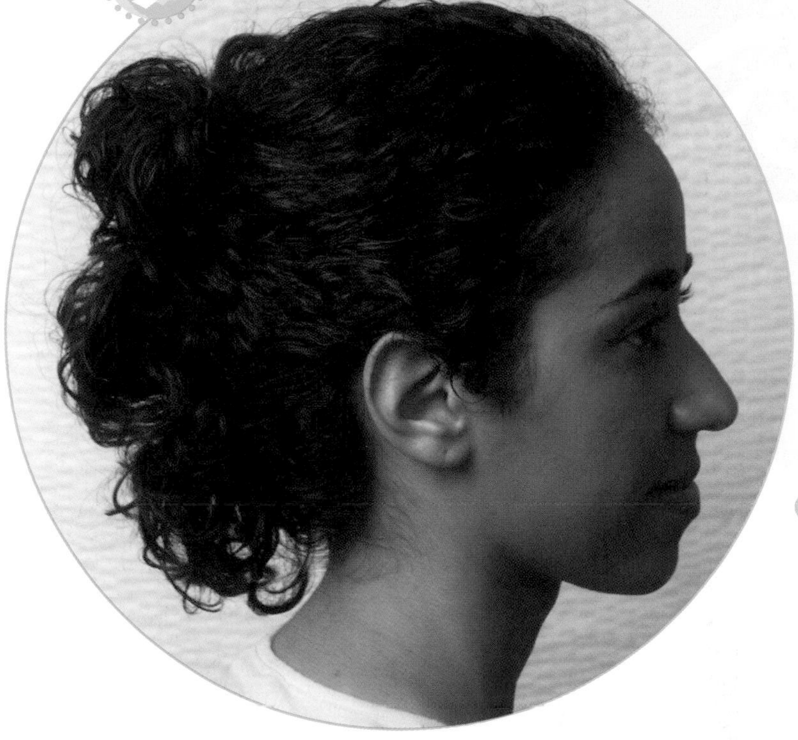

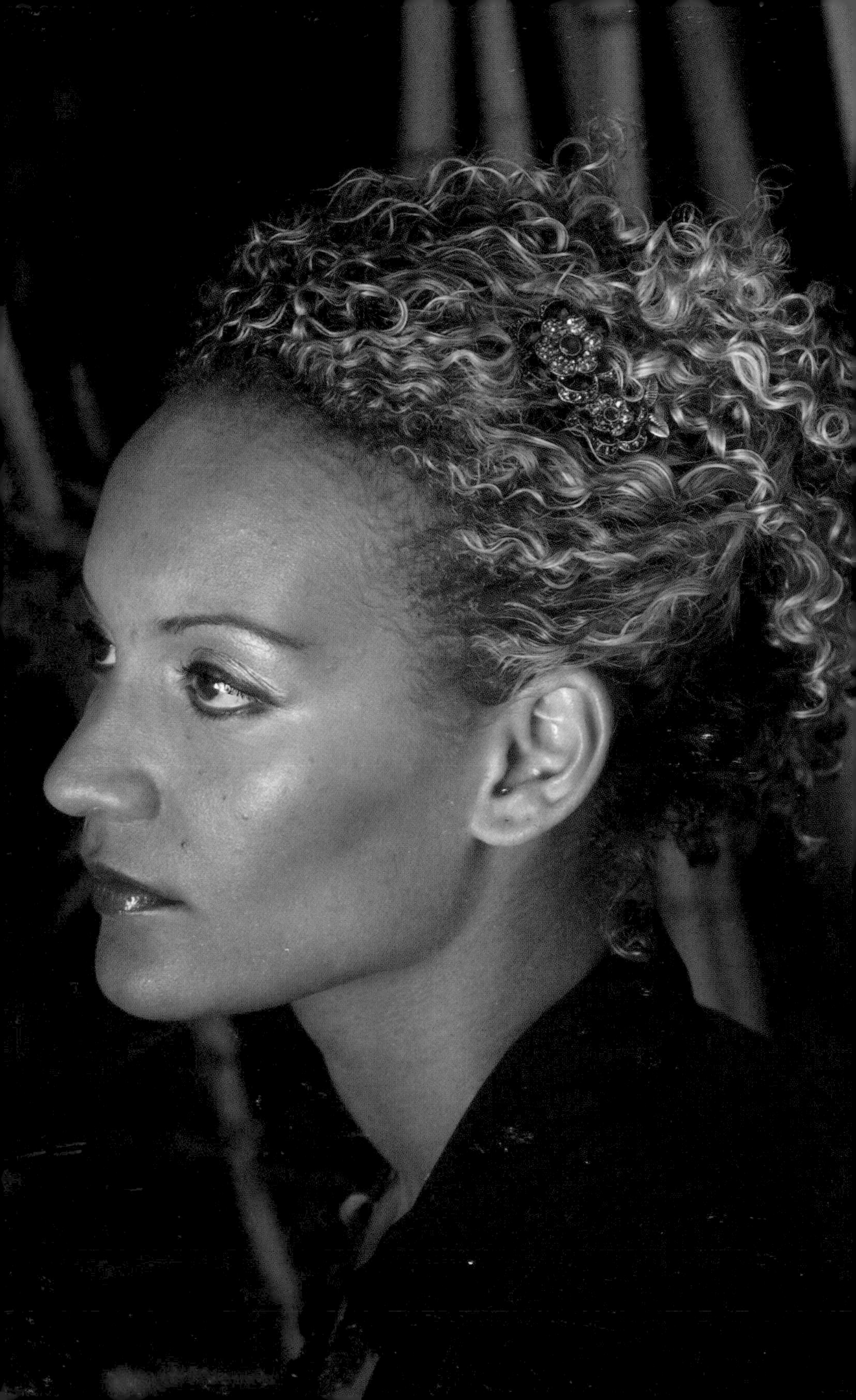

All Rolled Up

For shoulder length hair
or longer.

Rolling like the waves of the sea, this style connects everything together with a little curl in between.

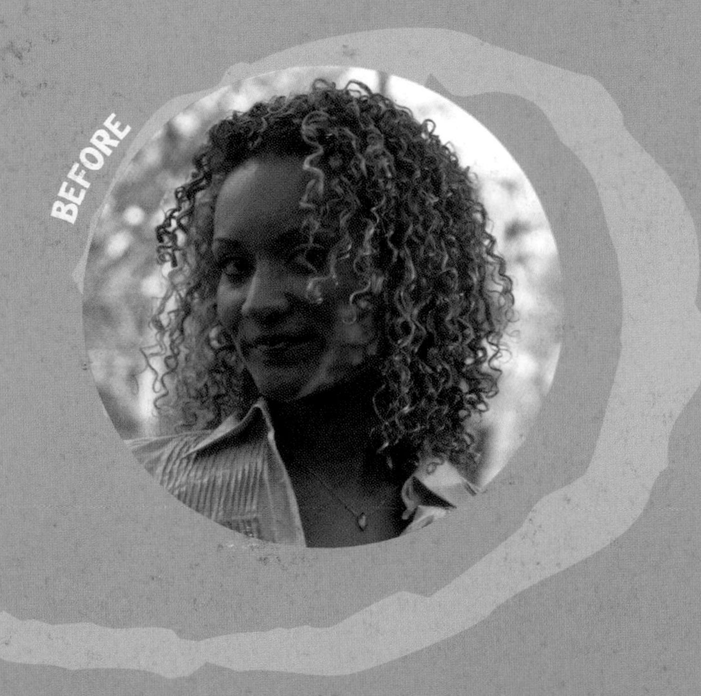

Step 1: At the crown of your head gather a two-inch by one-and-a-half-inch section of hair. Pull hair out from the crown of your head and hold with your left hand.

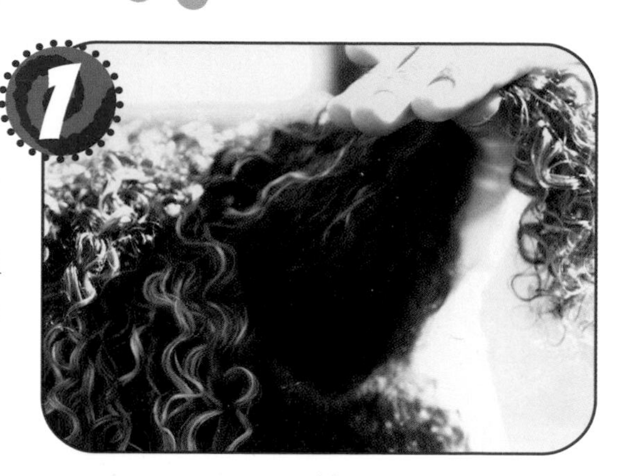

Step 2: Place your right hand at the crown with knuckles flat on your head, thumb pointing up. Gather the hair in the left hand and place over the right palm.

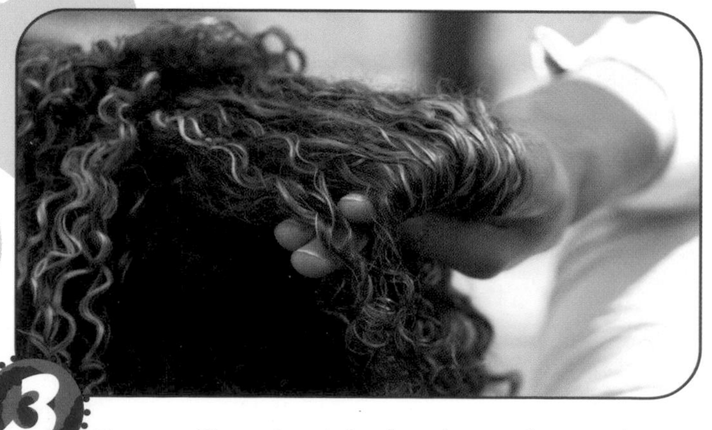

Step 3: Close the right thumb over hair and twist your right wrist down and then up. Your hand should automatically twist your hair into a barrel.

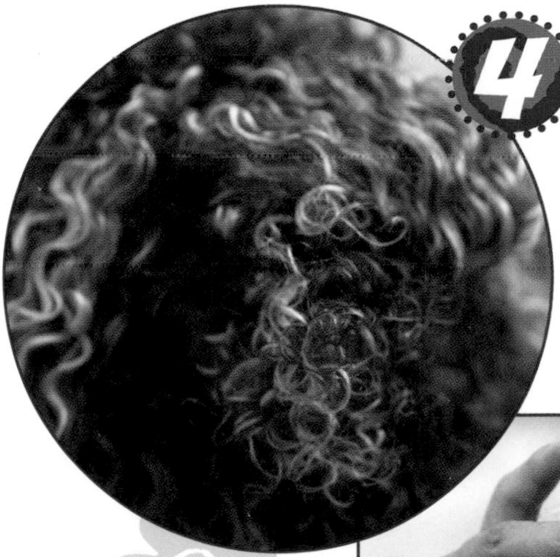

4

Step 4: Secure with a pin inside the barrel about where your thumb was. Your first barrel roll is complete. Don't forget to leave the ends of sectioned hair out.

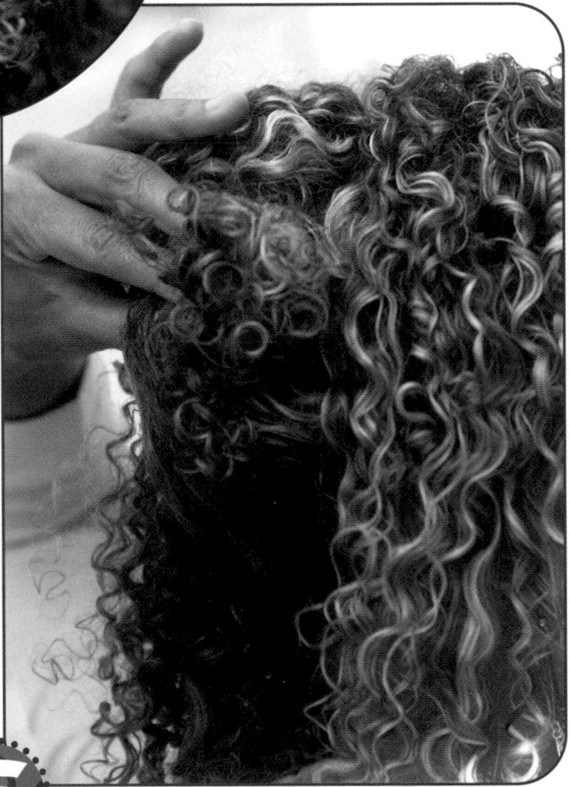

Note:
To pin the barrels, place a bobby pin at the edge of the barrel where the thumb of the twisting hand was located. Catch hair in the pin from the barrel and from the scalp while pushing the pin under the hair for coverage.

5

Step 5: Working in the back of the head, divide hair into three large sections. Each section should be about one-and-a-half-inches wide and approximately two inches long. The number of sections will vary depending upon the thickness of hair. One section at a time, create a barrel roll and secure.

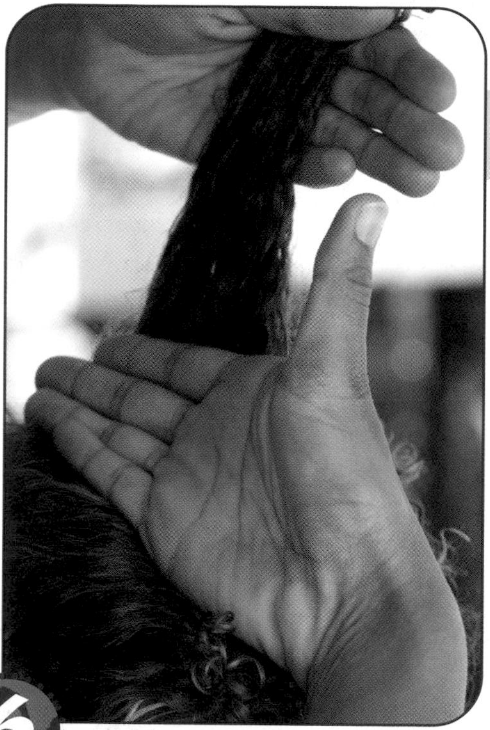

6

Step 6: Styling the back of your hair can be difficult. An alternative method is to hold the sectioned hair in your left hand. Place right hand right above the section of hair in the area where you want to form a barrel. Your right pinky finger and ring finger lay flat on your scalp. Place the section of hair into the palm of your hand and twist the right wrist up and around to create the barrel. Use this method for all the back sections. When completed, all the rolls should be touching, with the ends sticking out in between.

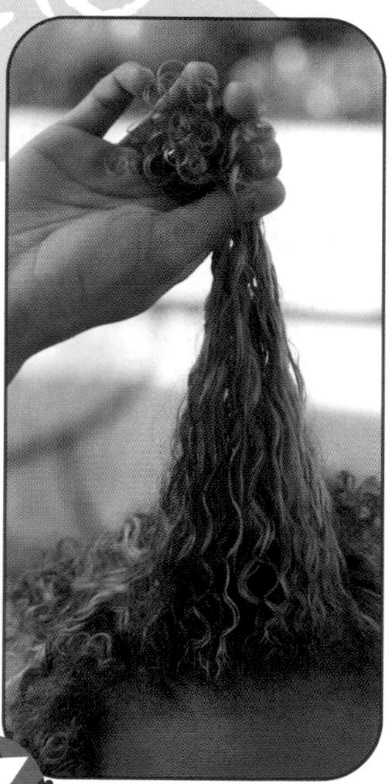

7

Step 7: After completing the back of your head, begin to style the front. Divide the portion of your hair into three or four sections. Make sure the sections are large, as shown in the picture. With the center section of hair, follow the directions in Step 2 to create a barrel roll and secure with pins.

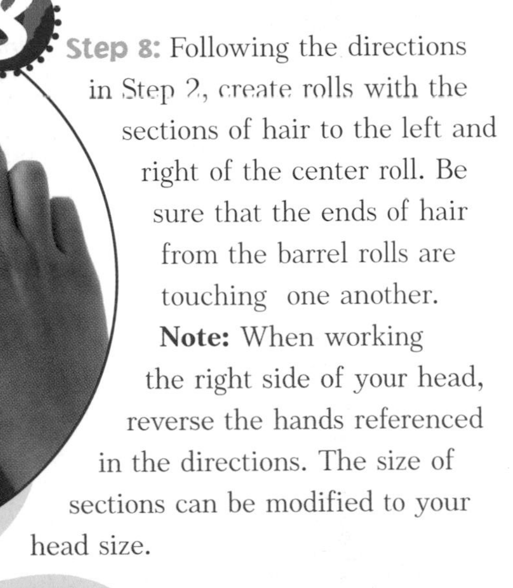

Step 8: Following the directions in Step 2, create rolls with the sections of hair to the left and right of the center roll. Be sure that the ends of hair from the barrel rolls are touching one another. **Note:** When working the right side of your head, reverse the hands referenced in the directions. The size of sections can be modified to your head size.

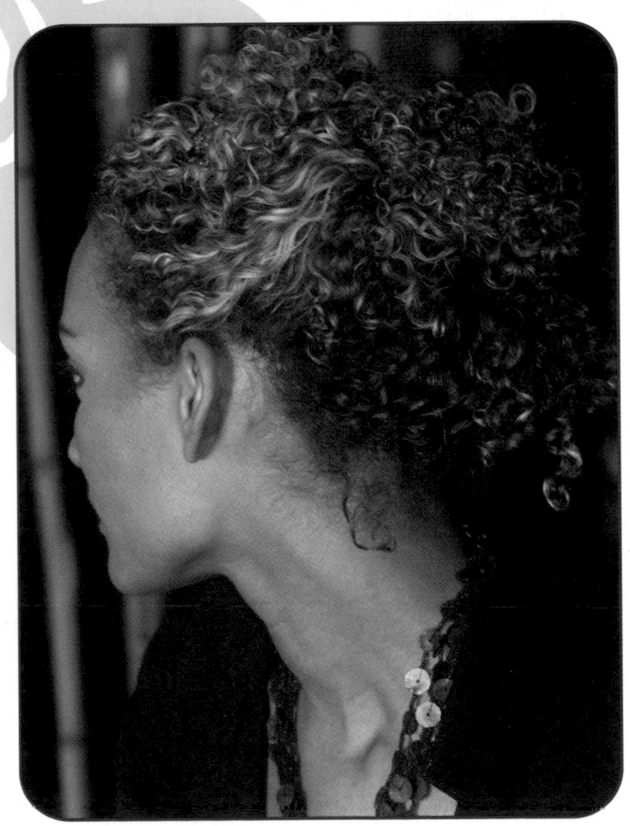

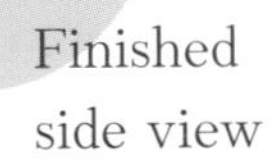

Finished side view

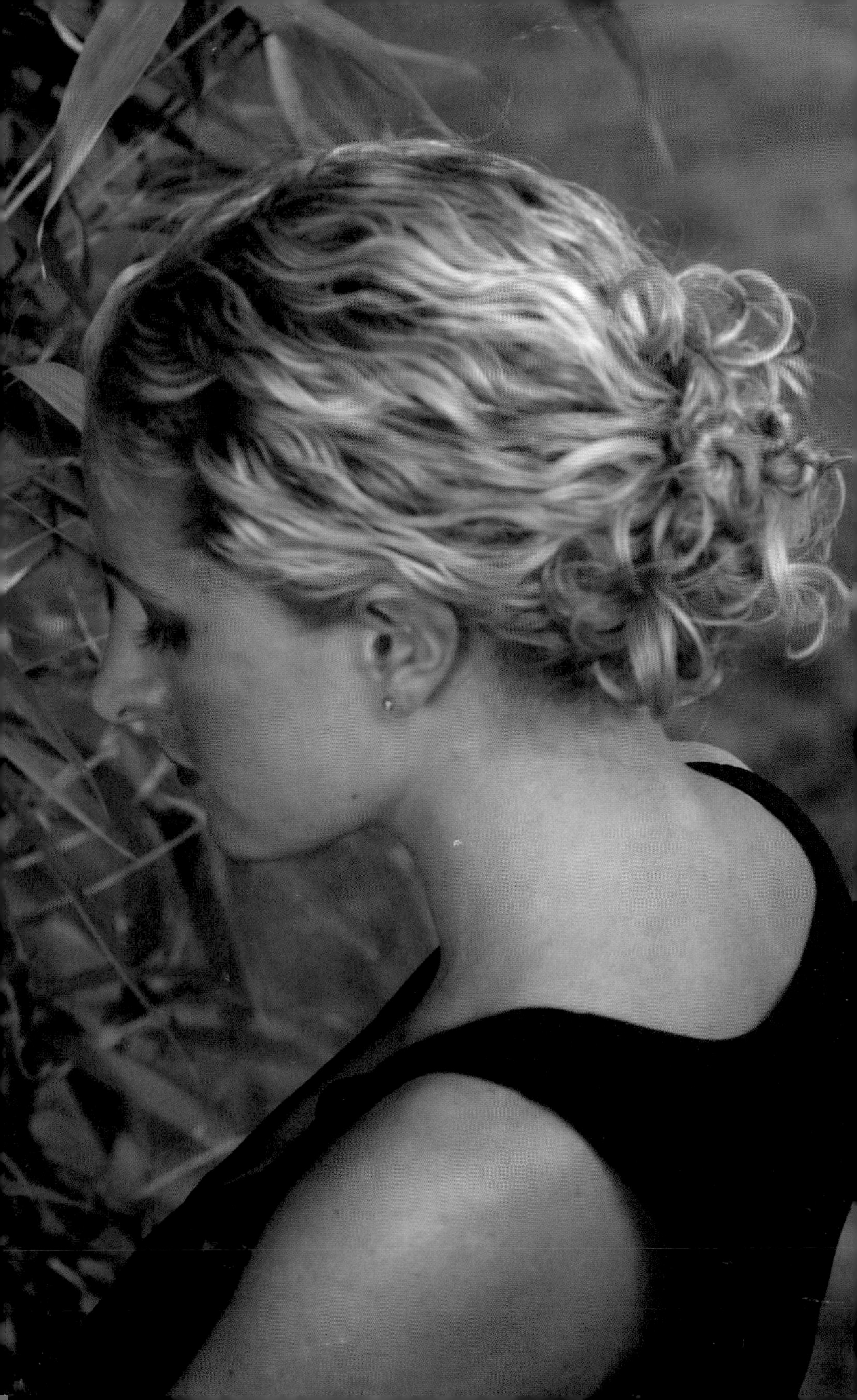

Nape Knots

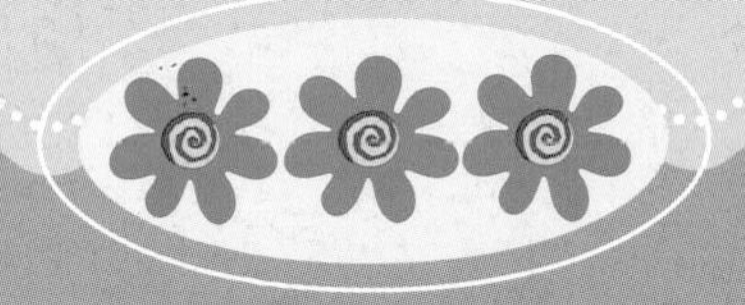

For shoulder length hair or longer. Long, layered hair is appropriate for this style.

A low cluster of curls, secured tightly at the nape of your neck. The perfect style for any occasion. Wear with the ends out or in for two separate but equally lovely looks.

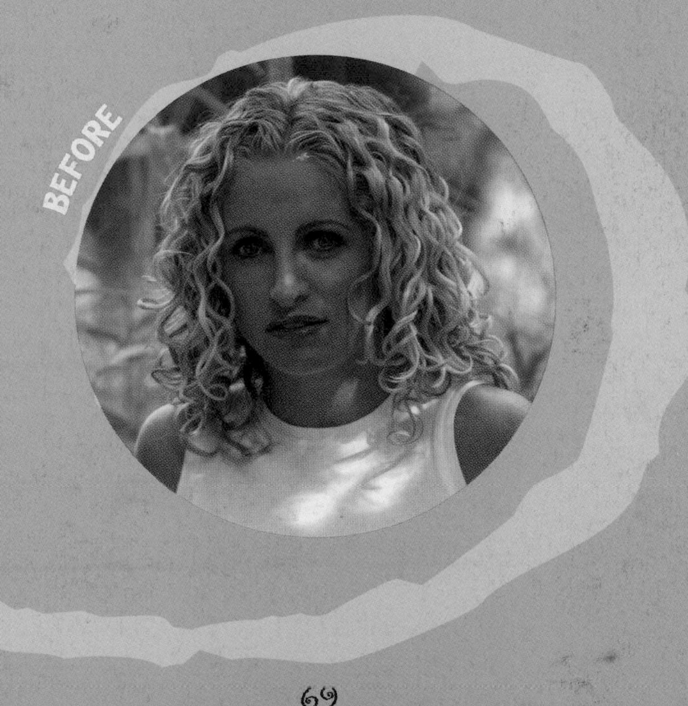

Step 1: Part hair according to your preference. Here we have created the zigzag part.

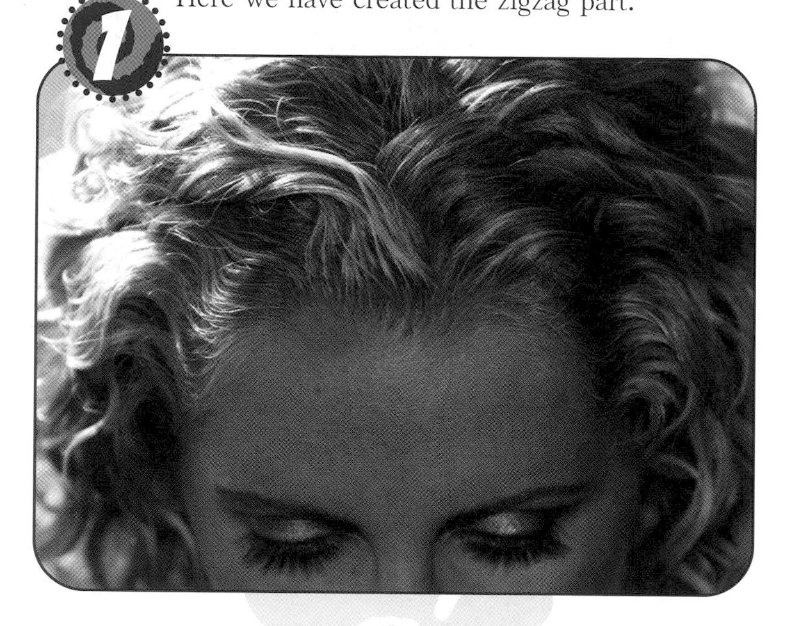

TIP:

To create a zigzag part, use the end of a rat-tail comb or other pointed object and carve a zigzag pattern through the hair, on the surface of the scalp from the hairline to the crown of your head. Once the comb has covered the length of the top of your head, lift up the hair with the comb and replace the comb with your fingers. Separate the two sides of hair and allow the hair to fall into the zigzag part.

This style takes practice, so do not become discouraged on your first try.

Step 2: Pull hair back into a low ponytail and secure with an elastic. The ponytail can be as tight or as loose as you like.

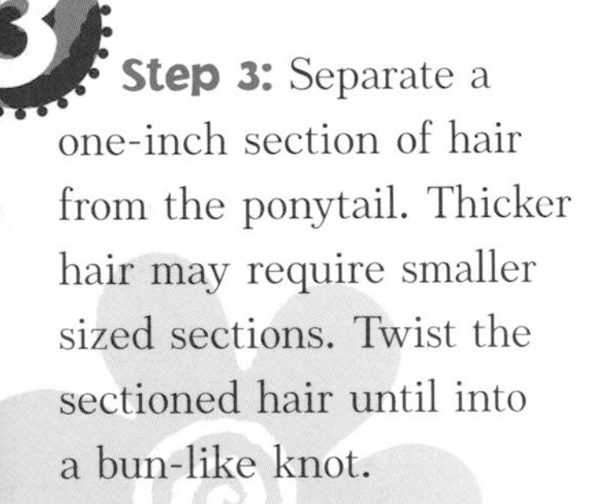

Step 3: Separate a one-inch section of hair from the ponytail. Thicker hair may require smaller sized sections. Twist the sectioned hair until into a bun-like knot.

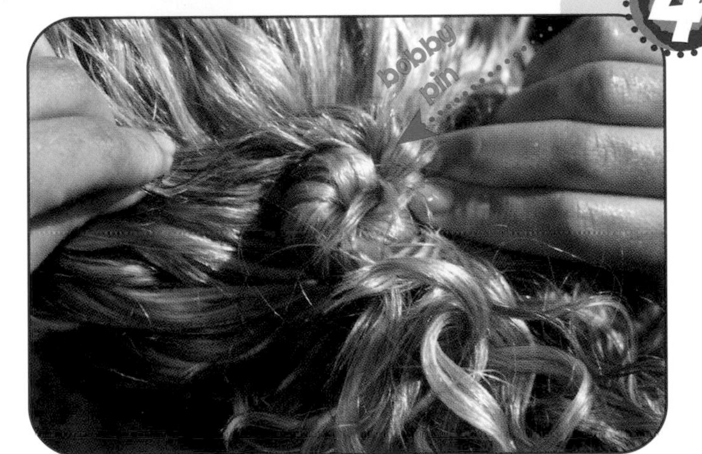

Step 4: Pin the knot to secure. Leave the ends of the sectioned hair out of the knot. Arrow indicates bobby pin placement.

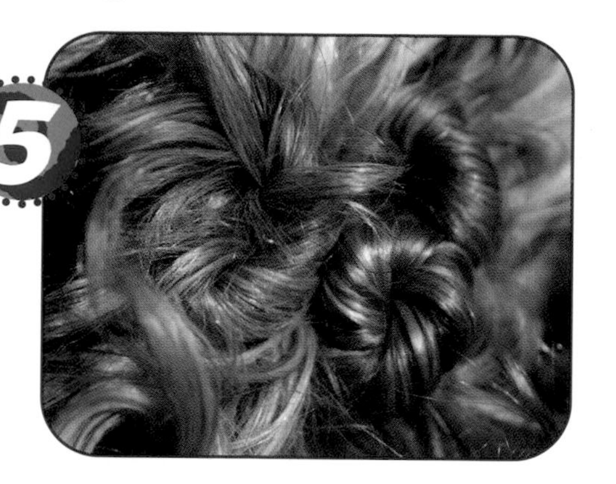

Step 5: Gather another section of hair from the ponytail same size as stated in Step 3. Twist sectioned hair down into a bun and secure.

6

Step 6: Work around the edges of the ponytail following the directions in Steps 4 and 5 until all the hair in the ponytail is twisted up and secured into small knotted buns.

7

Step 7: The final twists will be formed using the hair from the center section of the ponytail. Twist and secure the final pieces on top of the previously twisted knots to create a three dimensional effect.

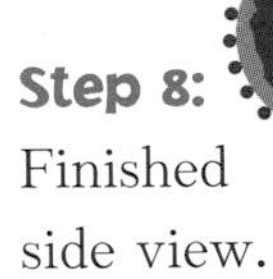

Step 8: Finished side view.

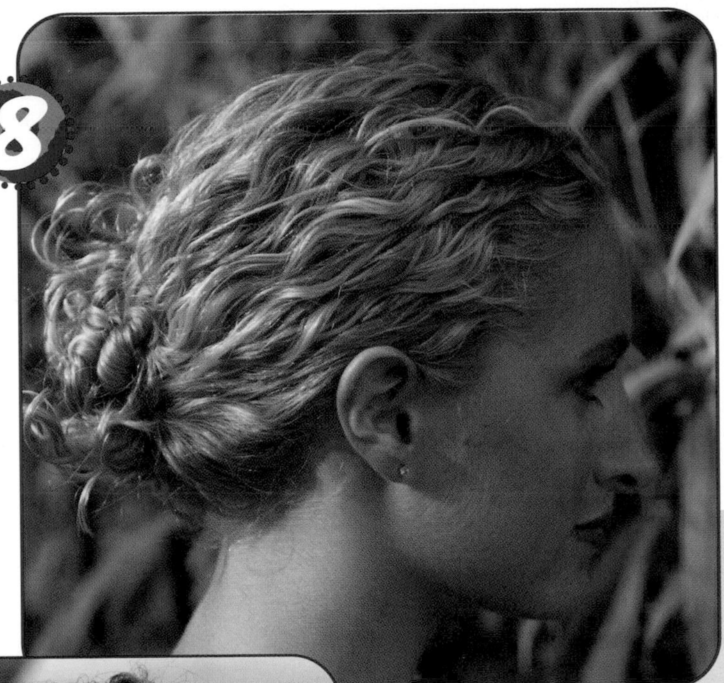

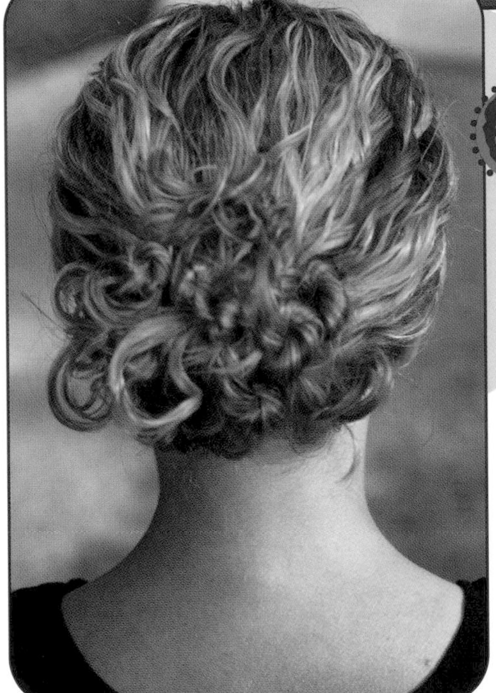

Step 9: Finished back. In this instance, the ends of the knotted buns are left out. However, twisting the ends into the buns creates a clean and polished look.

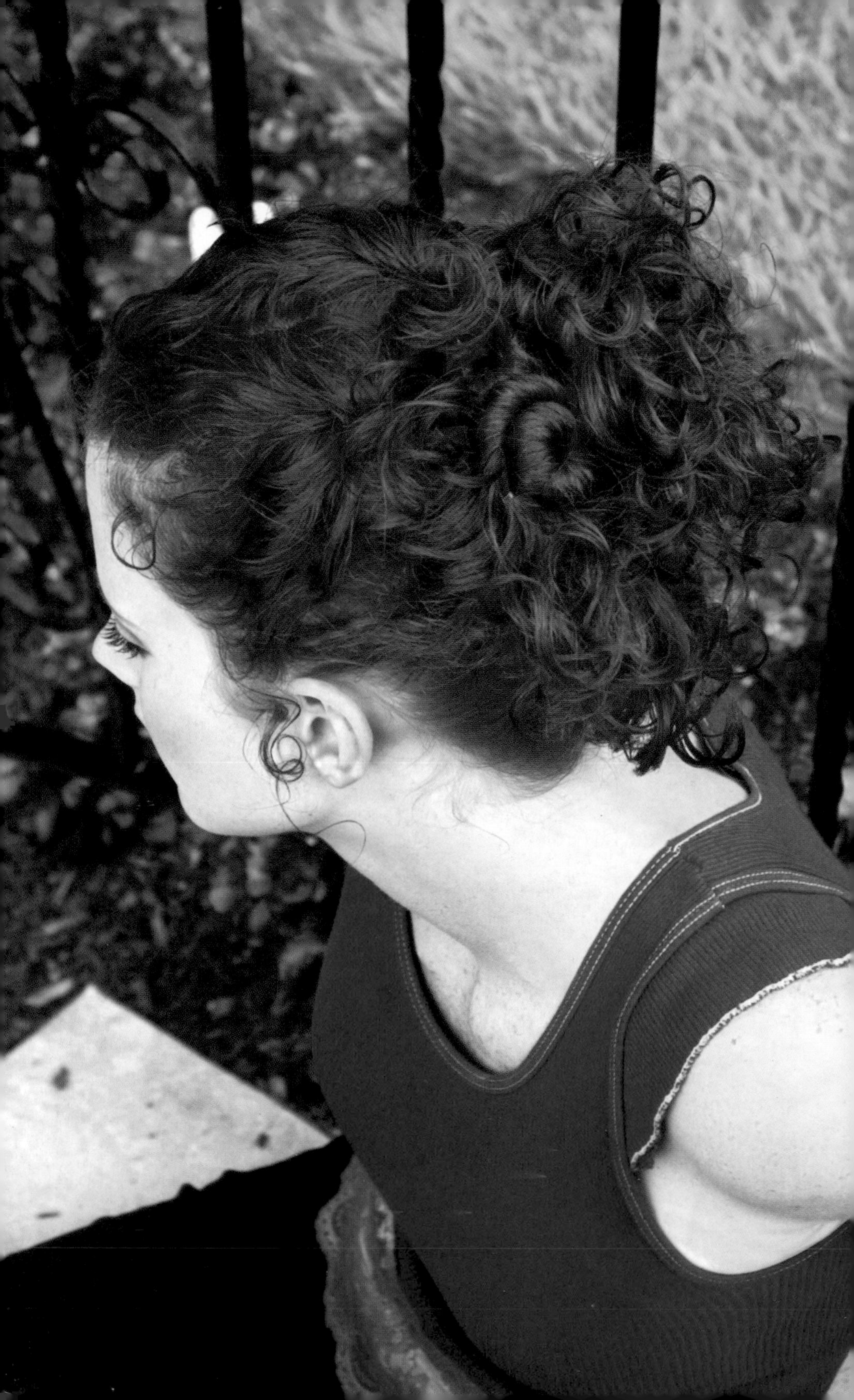

All Twisted Up

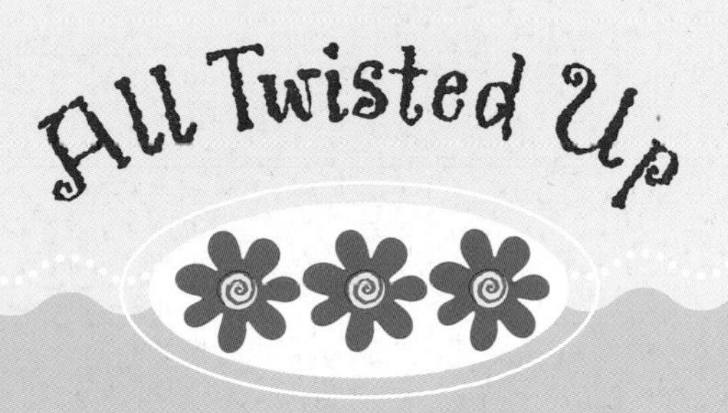

For shoulder length hair;
layers are acceptable.

Fun, flirtatious, functional! All words to describe this look! As noted by the three flowers, this look takes a little hair know-how; with a little practice you will succeed in mastering this look.

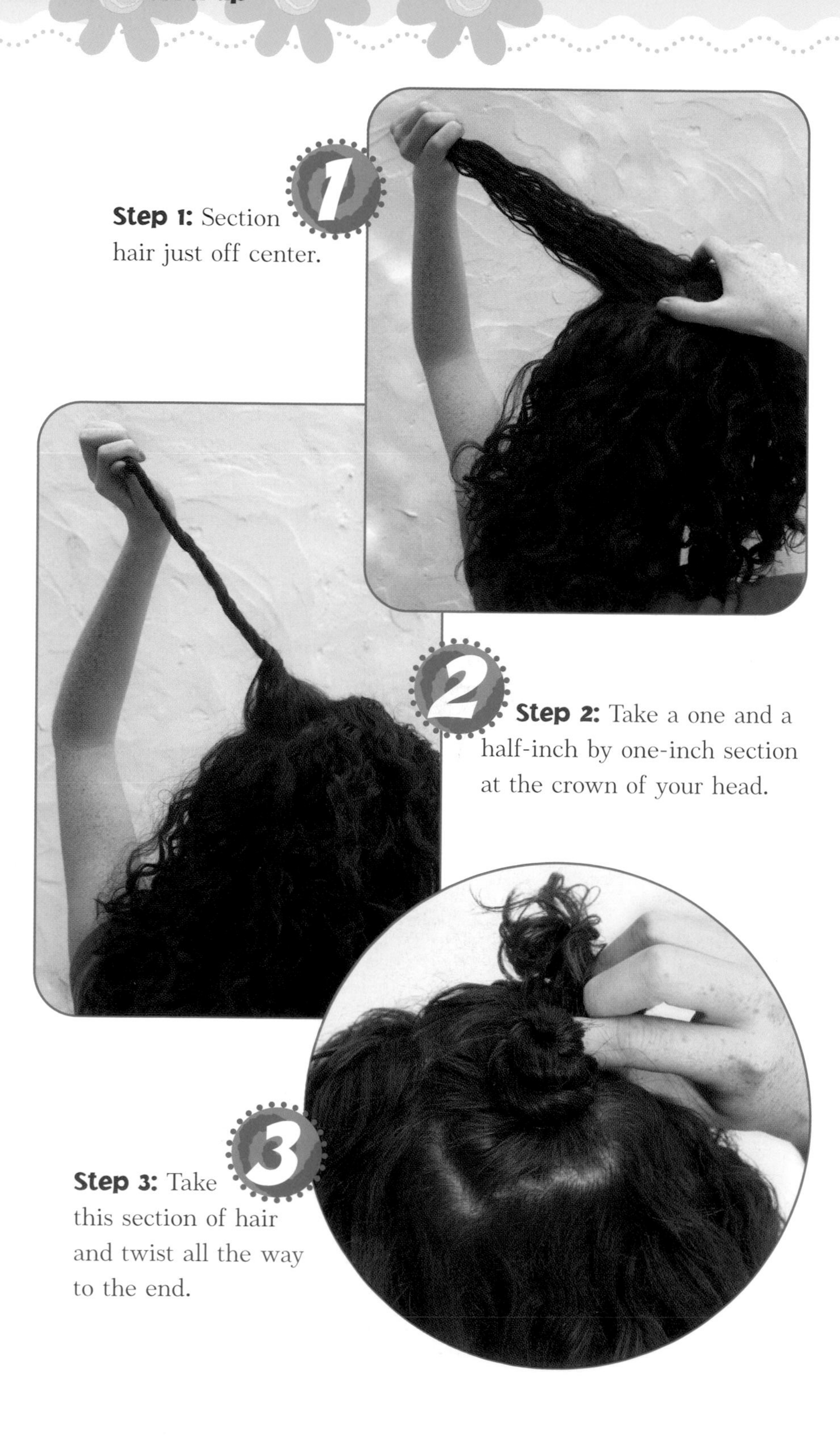

Step 1: Section hair just off center.

Step 2: Take a one and a half-inch by one-inch section at the crown of your head.

Step 3: Take this section of hair and twist all the way to the end.

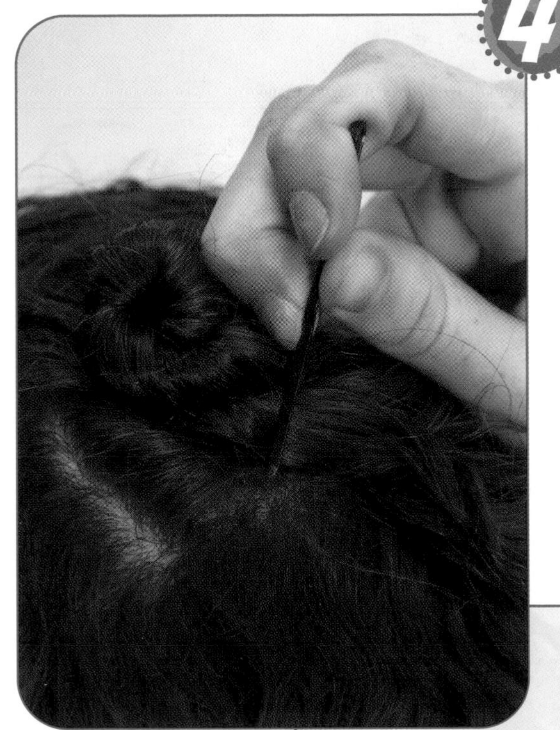

Step 4: Continue twisting this section of hair into a bun. Secure the bun in place by taking a bobby pin and straddling the end of the section of hair. Gently, push bobby pin to the scalp then direct it into the base of the bun.

Step 5: Take a two-inch section from behind the left ear to the top of the head and twist towards the previously secured bun at the crown.

Step 6: Mirror step 5 on the right side.

Step 7: You should have three buns now secured at the crown of the head with the ends left out.

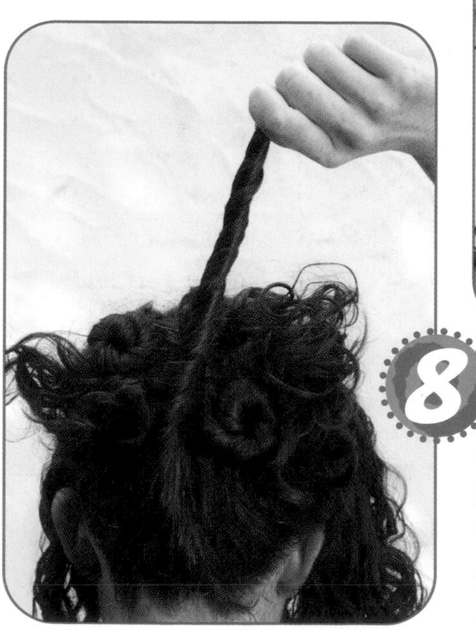

Step 8: Moving to the nape of the neck, divide the remaining hair in half from left to right. Take the left section, twist up and form a bun next to the existing buns and secure.

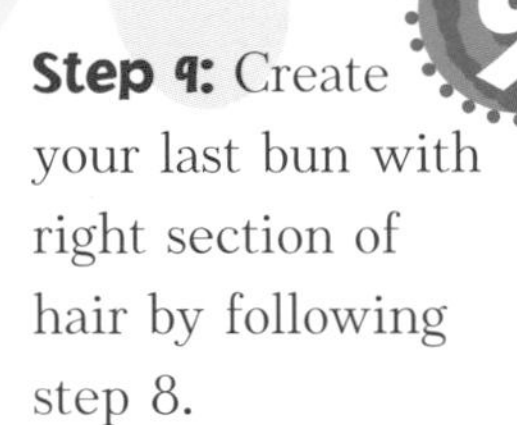

Step 9: Create your last bun with right section of hair by following step 8.

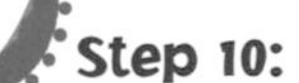

Step 10: Working on the front section of hair now, take all hair on the right side from the ear to the part and direct it back; twist this section and make a knot (refer to pages 76-77 to make a knot).

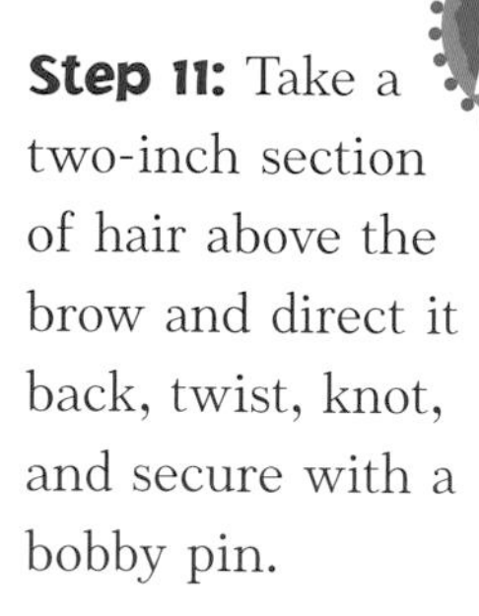

Step 11: Take a two-inch section of hair above the brow and direct it back, twist, knot, and secure with a bobby pin.

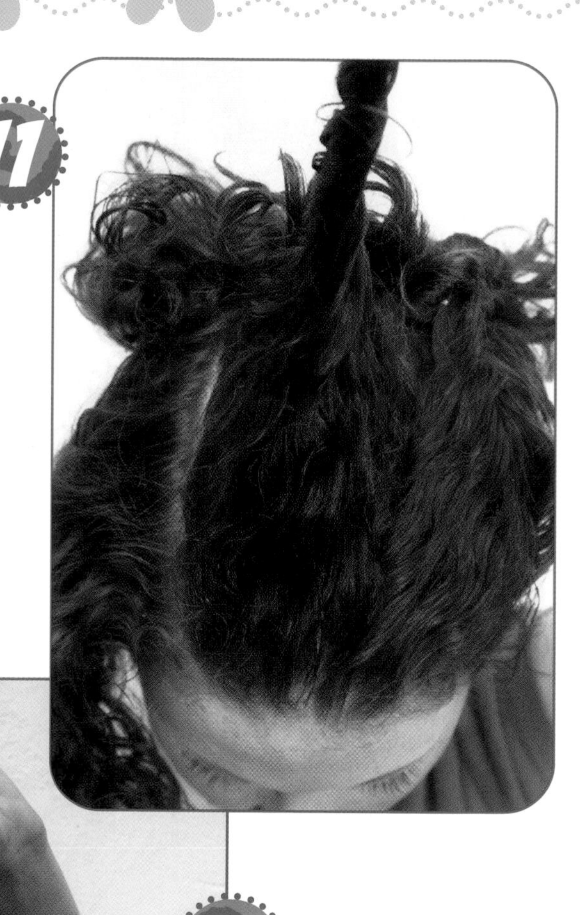

Step 12: Repeat step 10 on the left side of your hairline. Final twist is complete.

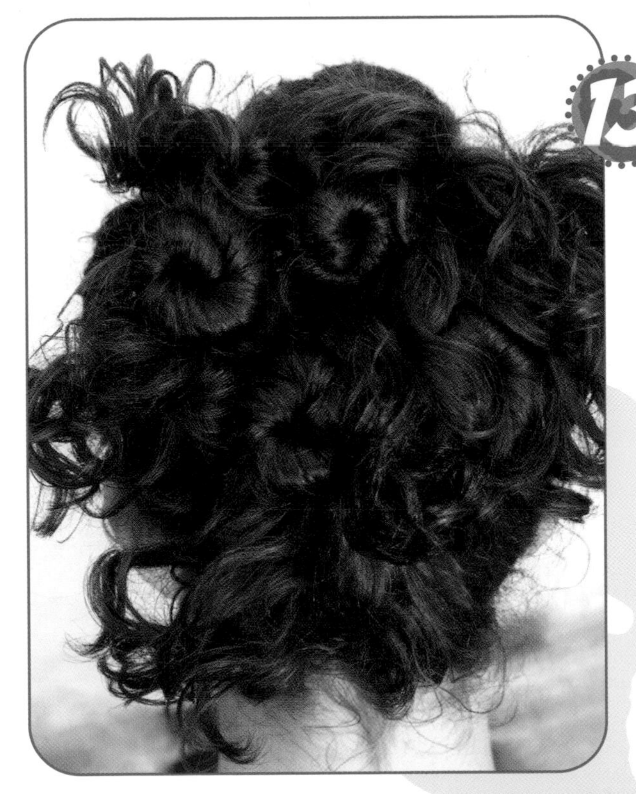

Step 13: Back view of finished look before fluffing the ends.

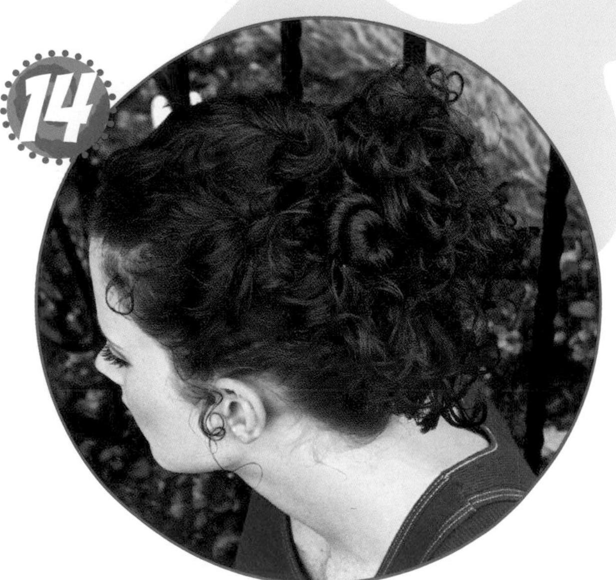

Step 14: Side view with the ends fluffed.

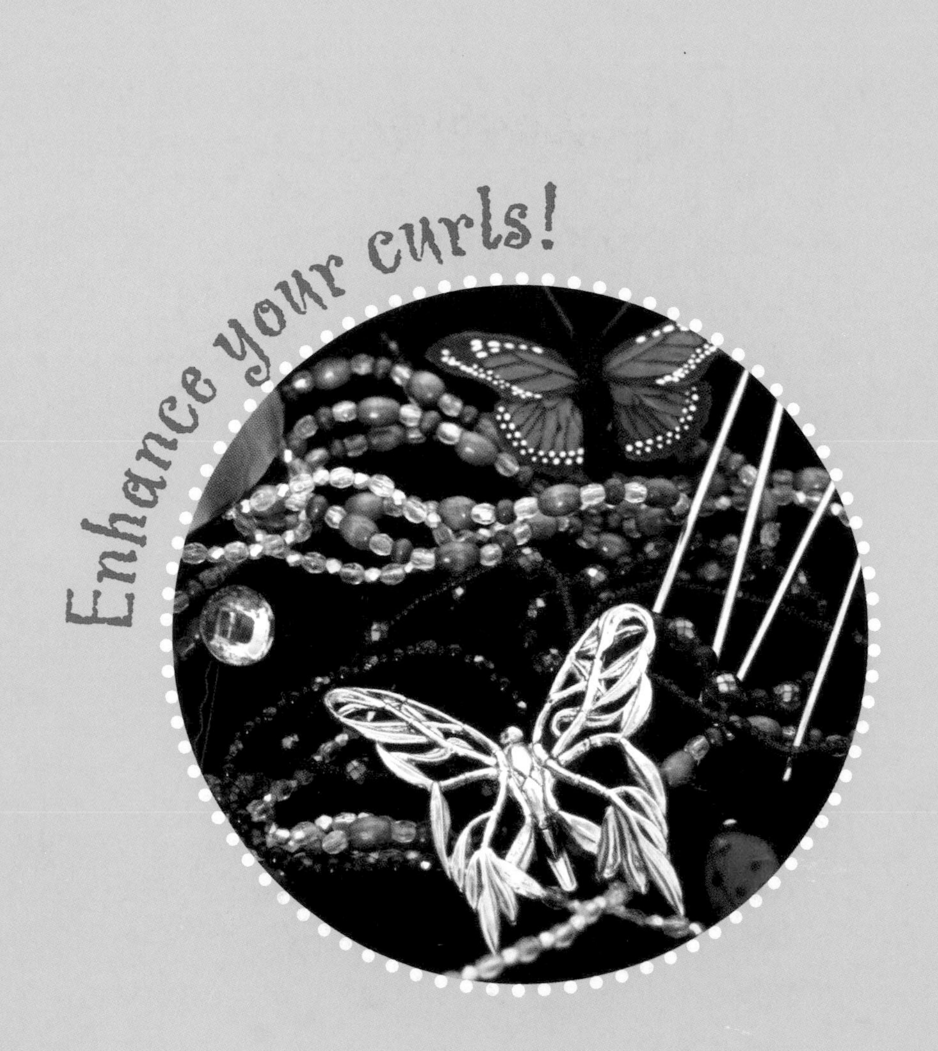
Enhance your curls!

Accessories

Add pizzazz!

Accessories can transform an everyday look into the illusion of a well-thought masterpiece of a hairstyle. Accessories can be found just about anywhere these days, from your local mall to the craft store, and they vary in price. With a little creativity you can make your own hair accessory; in fact, I show you how to make your own in the next two pages and also give you some tips to make a beaded bracelet into a hair accessory.

• At your local craft store in the floral department they have a selection of artificial insects such as ladybugs, bumble bees, or butterflies. These sometimes have wire attached already so all you would do is cut the wire down to about two and a half inches long, then hook the end so it won't slide out of your hair when you move your head around. Then, slide in place to any of the styles you've just learned how to do. If your accessory of choice does not come with wire then you will need a hot glue gun and a bobby pin. The bobby pin should be as close to your hair color as possible. Put a dot of glue on the closed side of the bobby pin, not the side that opens. Refer to picture above for placement. Then simply place your object onto the glue and allow to dry. Here we used ladybug on the end of a bobby pin.

• Another trick is to get a button you like so long as it has the looped back and not button holes. The loop needs to be big enough to get one leg of the bobby pin through.

Simply open the bobby pin, slide the button over one leg of the bobby pin until you reach the bend and stop. The button should stay at the bent end. Now it is ready to accentuate your style.

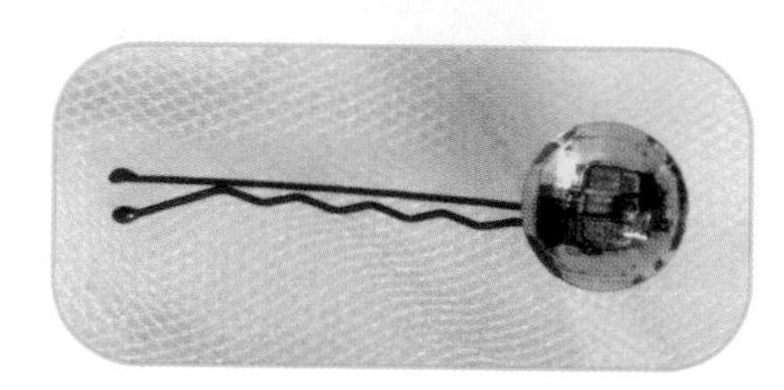

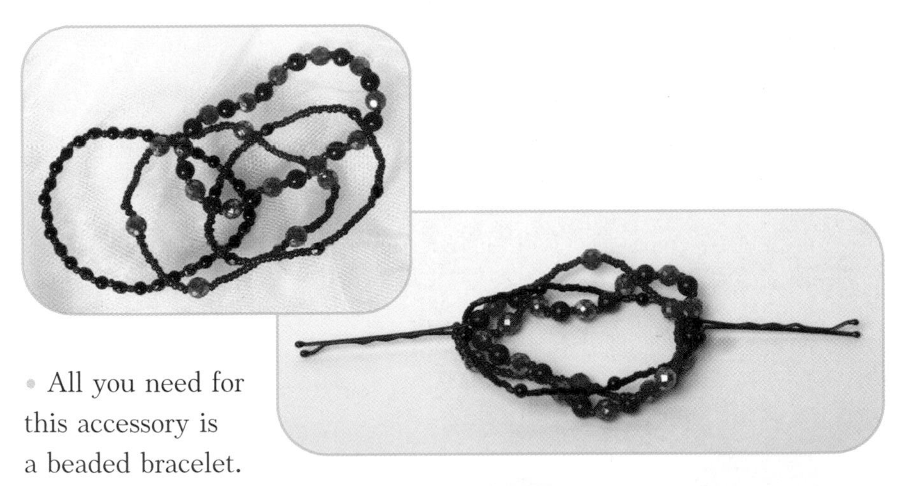

All you need for this accessory is a beaded bracelet. Take two bobby pins; lay the bracelet flat on a table, place one bobby pin on either side of the bracelet. (See photo above.) Now insert into hair. For placement, put one bobby pin in on one side of the twist and insert the other bobby pin on the other side of the twist, making sure the bracelet is hanging with a little sag in the middle rather than pulled really tight. This looks best with multiple bracelets.

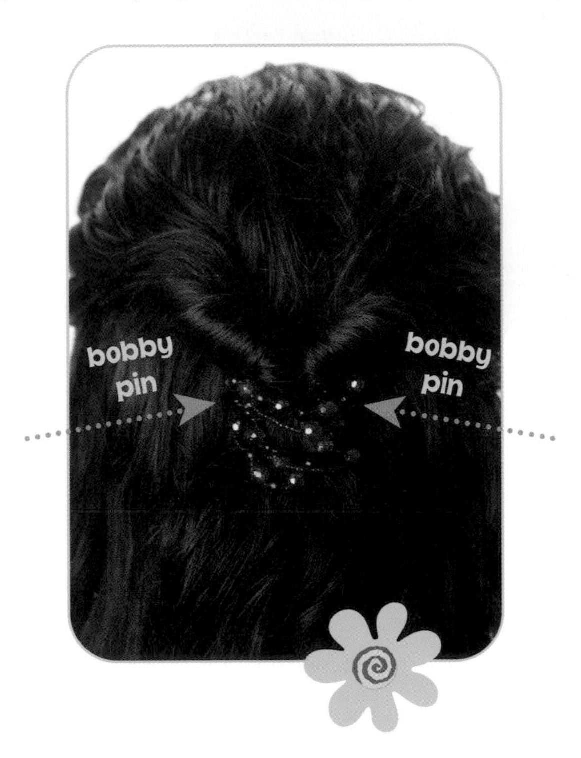

Secure your curls!

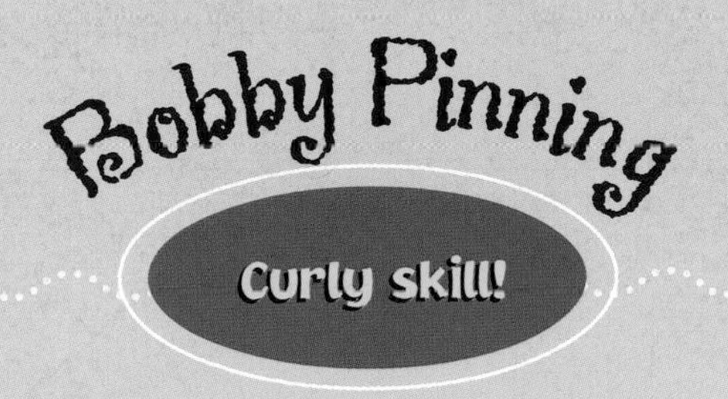

The key to many of these styles in this book is bobby pinning. When you know how to bobby pin properly, the styles are endless. You can even start creating your own.

Two important qualities to have when securing with bobby pins are obscurity and security. It is very important to make sure your bobby pin is not seen. They are not meant to be used as accessories unless decorated as such. The standard brown and black bobby pins are intended to secure your style in place, so visually we want to see as little as possible. Secondly, security. If you don't have security you won't have peace of mind. You don't want to worry that half-way through the day a pin may come loose and your twist will uncoil, leaving a look of Medusa for all to see!

Here are some tips to security and obscurity. With practice and patience, you can create any style.

Making your pins camouflaged starts by choosing pins the same color as your hair. The size of the bobby pin should be considered next. If your hair is very thick and/or coarse you will need the longer, thicker bobby pins. They're about two inches long. This will stay put more easily with thicker hair density. The standard size bobby pin should work just fine for less dense hair. Most grocery stores carry these, but if not, try your local beauty supply store. You can find bobby pins in a box in large amounts at your beauty supply store also. You may want to get a large supply because you'll want to wear your hair up all the time now that you know how to style it up!

Securing a bobby pin will take some practice so don't get discouraged.

Here are a few examples of how to bobby pin:

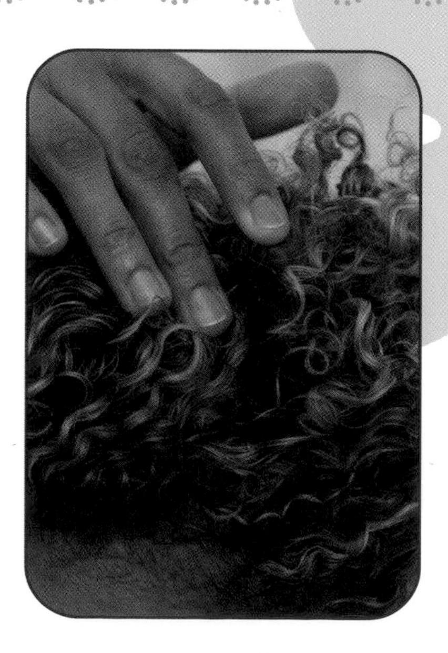

- **To secure the barrel roll,** start by pushing the bobby pin straight down until it touches the scalp of your head, then direct the pin into the barrel.

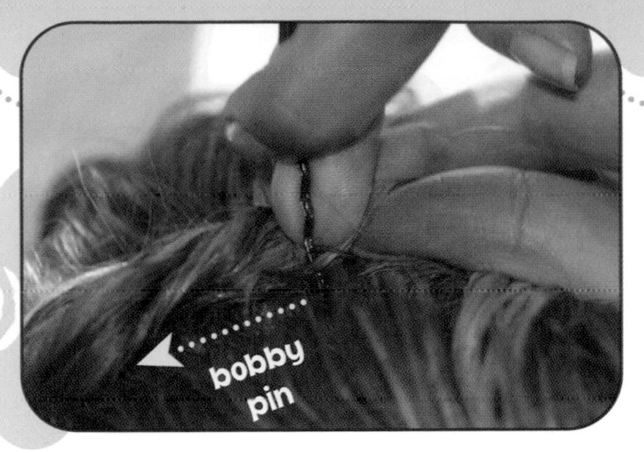

• **To straddle a twist,** start by separating the "legs" of the bobby pin one leg on either side of the twist. For a large twist you may need to put one leg through the middle of the twist and the other leg on the outside. If your bobby pin does not stay with it in the middle your twist may be too thick and you may need to divide this twist into two twists. After the pin is straddled, direct the pin up the twist, going against the direction the hair is moving.

• **This is an example of how NOT to secure a bun.** Here the bobby pin is too close to the surface and not hidden well.

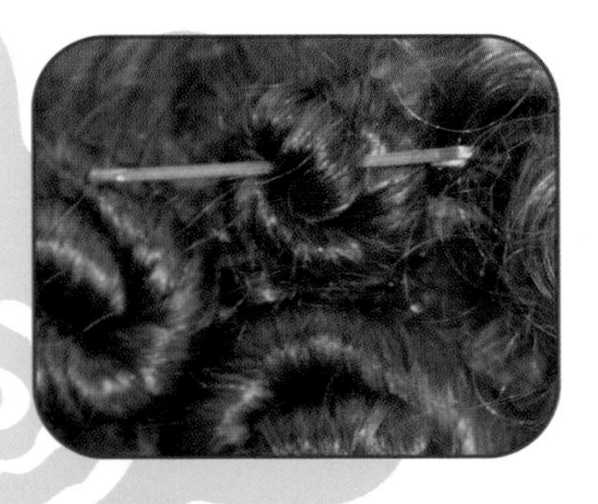

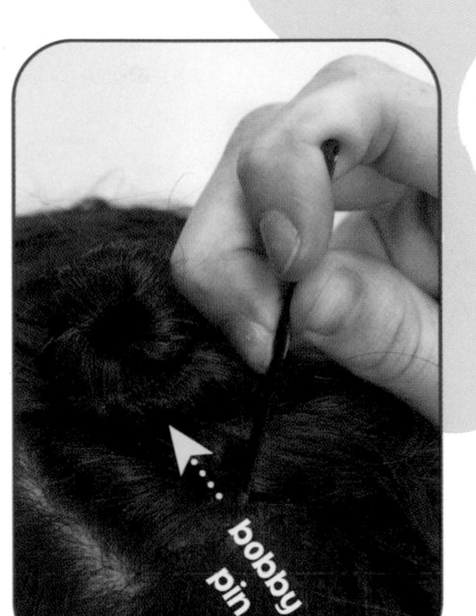

• **This picture shows how to properly secure a bun.** Start by straddling the end of the already twisted section of hair. Push straight onto the scalp and direct the bobby pin into the bun, staying close to the scalp and trying to weave the pin through the bottom on the bun.